Make The Hood Healthy Again

Asa Lockett

With a foreword from Rafa Wright

Plug'd Media 2021
Published in 2021 in Detroit, Michigan
ISBN: 978-1-7375671-0-3

"<u>We are losing more people to sweets than to the street</u>." More than any act of violence done to us either internally or externally, poor health is single handedly the greatest murderer in the hood. From obesity, to diabetes, to heart disease, to hypertension, various forms of cancer, and other ailments, we are dying at rate like no other time in history. If our villages do not reclaim its health, I do not know how much longer we will have.

Growing up, I cannot remember listening to music promoting a healthy lifestyle. We only heard about how to get and keep money. More than this, our culture taught us many of our common unhealthy living habits we hold as standards today – poor diet, drug and alcohol overconsumption, hypersexual activity, misogyny, self-hate, and violence. Most of all, farming and gardening, home cooked meals, and grocery stores have been replaced with corporate entities that puts profit over health through laboratory foods. We are so separated from our true selves. Its time to reconnect.

I talk about financial independence a lot, but what good is money when your dead before you can genuinely enjoy it? We live fast because we never know when things will be over. Do we think about what we do to bring about our own demise? Wake up, have chips and juice for breakfast, a cheeseburger deluxe with chili and cheese on the fries for lunch, and a #1 at Wendy's for dinner, all with lots of weed and lean in the middle of each course. Then you wonder why your legs cannot fit in those $1,000 designer skinny jeans, and your belly is holding up your $10,000 diamond chain. About time we reach our financial prime, we are on our death bed. This cannot be life, at all.

At the end of the day, our communities must prioritize health the same we prioritize financial security. In fact, we would not have financial security without our physical, mental, and spiritual health being aligned. So, our health should always be main priority.

We are perhaps the unhealthiest group in the world. Much of this is because of systematic racism which has limited, restricted, or outright eliminated opportunities and options for us to live healthy lives, like proper healthcare, nutritional education, healthy food access, gyms and fitness facilities, and mental health services. Our immune systems are so beat down, our mental health is so deteriorated, and we are so disconnected from the universe that many of us will not survive.

I want good health, and wealth for everyone. More than that, I need everyone to realize the opportunities that are in front of us. Technology is making it easier to produce, transport, store, and share. The ball is truly in our courts to ball out, the right way. The author of this piece, Asa Lockett, and me are coming together to take advantage of what we know we have to present to you a full embodiment of wellness so that we can reconnect to our true selves. We are gods and goddesses walking on this beautiful planet, only if we believe we are and only if we do the necessary work to manifest that reality. No virus, or system formed against us shall prosper if we come together, unlearn, re-learn, apply pressure, and build the foundation

I met Asa years ago and have always respected his work. I really believe in his guidance as a healer. After reading what he wrote in this work, you will believe in him like I do. I am blessed to now call this God my brother, and you will be blessed after reading this.

Make The Hood Healthy Again is a work aimed to equip you with the knowledge to achieve and maintain optimum physical, mental, sexual, and spiritual health. More than that, Make The Hood Healthy Again is a piece that champions balance between the mind, body, spirit, and universe. Most of all, Make The Hood Healthy Again is another encouraging work that strives to show ghetto babies across this nation, and world, they have the power to mold their realities into whatever they wish, that heaven on earth is achievable if you pour into the right temples, in the right order, with the right balance, for the right reasons.

The concept of a better inner-city America starts with

health. The healthier we are, the wealthier we will be. Some recurring concepts in this book are:

- Your community/environment affects your overall health.
- Being mindful of who is in charge of "healing" us.
- Food is everything – medicine, pleasure, and history/culture.
- Your body is a machine that requires a balanced preventative maintenance in order to properly function – nutrition, physical activity, mental activity, and rest.
- More of the body, it is a temple that houses your soul which has some requirements to manifest.
- Overconsumption will kill you.
- Physical, mental, and spiritual balance is what will bring about optimum health.
- We are all connected to everything

In this book, Asa drops gems on:
- Food – Where, when, how to eat?
- Hydration – What, when, how to drink?
- Rest – When, where, how to rest?
- Mental health – eliminating barriers in the mind.
- Spiritual health – how to channel the universe and our inner God/Goddess to manifest all that we desire.

The mind is only as good as the temple it is in. Health is wealth. The time is now to get healthy so that we can fight the good/hood fight in this world. I want to thank Asa for allowing me to be present in this project. I hope that the words written here reach everyone safely and last for generations into the future.

One thing to note about this work: Asa is doing so much of the heavy lifting here. I am providing commentary to all the gems he is dropping here. At best, look at me at the moderator to this groundbreaking piece of literature. While Asa is baking the cake, I'll be adding the icing to it. I hope y'all are ready to transform. All love!!!

– Rafa Wright

#MakeTheHoodHealthyAgain

Table of Contents

Ch.1: Make The Hood Healthy Again

The purpose of this writing is not to dictate one's food selections nor is it to instruct one on what is right or wrong in regards to his or her diet. This book was written with the intention of reminding the reader how we work and how to manifest the best version of ourselves. The desire of the authors here is to empower the reader with a holistic approach to caring for both the mental and physical bodies and the environment around us. Sadly many of us can only take our history back to what we were taught about slavery. We are ignorant of our global excellence spanning over millions of years. The truth is that the primal power that allowed for us to seed and civilize the planet has never left us. Even though we seem to be getting further away from our greatness, this too is an illusion. As the pressure increases, the universe has its own plans. Let us take a look into how we can bring that divine condition back into our modern day homes and neighborhoods.

Sadly, many of us can only take our history back to what we were taught about slavery. We are ignorant of our global excellence spanning over hundreds of thousands of years. ***The truth is that the primal power that allowed for us to seed and civilize the planet has never left us.*** Even though we seem to be getting further away from our greatness, this too is an illusion. As the pressure increases, the universe has its own plans. Let us take a look into how we can bring that divine condition back into our modern-day homes and neighborhoods.

Are You Really Healthy?

We often use the word heal without having a true understanding of what the word entails. Many people will offer up their opinions on the matter however in its original context it means to *return* or to restore something back to its original state. A clear example of this is something we are all familiar with. Let's say a person cuts himself or herself somehow and a visible scar is present. After a week or so they may notice that their skin looks the same as it did before the cut because the body is always seeking to heal and has the capacity to restore itself back to normal. This however is only an example of healing on a very dense and physical level. We are capable of healing on deeper and more subtle levels as well. As a matter of fact the internal portions of the person are much more important than what we see on the outside. True healing takes place when we choose to align our attention and actions with the natural order of the universe. This is a very sacred and personal journey as we all have our own trials and experiences to learn from and triumph over. True health encompasses the entire being of the person so if one looks pristine on the outside but has imbalances internally then he or she does not qualify to be called healthy. Understand that the physical body is a container and a vehicle for the being inside. It can be called an extension of the being but should not be confused with the essence of the person occupying it. This simple change in perspective will save a lot of people from unnecessarily running into problem after problem from trying so called solutions that only address the densest parts of the body while completely ignoring the spirit beneath it. We tend to get in the way of the healing process due to our modern day thinking and our not so productive habits.

Unfortunately we are taught by the mainstream educational systems to address the physical body as our primary target when it comes to improving our health. The physicists then go ahead to teach us that the physical world as we know it only makes up about four percent of the universe. The main methods used to address our health concerns are medication and surgery, both of which leave us in even more of a detrimental state after their "services." The medications are not only incapable of healing us. They each have their own set of side effects that show up after usage that all call for yet another form a medication to "save the day." Before you know it, we are expected to take anywhere from five to ten different forms of medication before we die. What makes this matter completely unacceptable is the fact that these medications are not designed to work in concert with one another and this of course results in a web of confusion inside our bodies. The surgeries, which cost us even more money, leave us physically deformed and unable to perform our duties on earth in peak performance. They tend to go for the less popular glands or organs when this of course has its own domino effect on the rest of the body. For example, some people allow the doctors to remove their pancreas, which serves as the home for intuition while others allow the removal of their spleen, which plays a crucial role in the distribution of solar forces throughout the body. Matters like this will continue to happen until we begin to assume responsibility over our well-being. No doctor should know more about your body than you. When we see an increase in accountability for how we govern ourselves, we will see a decrease in the bold and brutal practices carried out today by the hands of those who profess to have your best interest in mind. We say that the human body is the living temple of God but we sure don't act like it.

In order to address our health in a more appropriate manner, it is important that we begin with acknowledging where the body comes from in the first place. Even though it is physically developed in our mother's womb, we need to go back even further or higher to get a clearer understanding of what we are dealing with. Keep in mind that this is the world of reflections and what things look like. Our true nature is much more subtle and behind the scenes. We have scientific evidence now proving that essentially we are composed of stardust. The ancient Egyptians said that before the beginning and before existence existed there were the waters of nu. Mind you, astrophysicists and those leading the so called quantum research today are still baffled and scratching their heads trying to understand our cosmic origins. They use terms like the big bang to describe what our ancestors called ptah which was understood as the conversion point between "nothing" to something or the mind making itself manifest. They use terms like dark matter to describe what our ancestors called the waters of nu, which was understood as the cosmic clay that could be molded or shaped into anything in existence. Throughout the course of this book we will show and prove how profound and glorious our ancestors were and how uneducated we have been in regards to them.

According to field theory, all planets, stars, and galaxies are torus energy systems defined by their central black hole and these black holes are points of singularity (zero point or stillness). Johannes Kepler, the famous German astronomer, mathematician, and astrologer from the 1500s, referred to black holes as "unified fields and places where infinite potential lies waiting to accommodate any act or audience." You the reader are technically a black hole with an opening at the mouth and another at the anus. How does this affect your capacity to heal?

We were taught that we are human in the sense that we are powerless in comparison to "God" and the more dynamic forces present in the universe but we are constantly being shown thru science and other mediums how profound and mind blowing we are if we simply just were to put the pieces together. This is a perfect example of why holistic learning is important and why you should make it a point to learn how to think for yourself as opposed to just accepting the perspectives that the media and the mainstream educational systems bombard us with. You have no plugs whereby you need to attach yourself to something externally like a phone charger or a television set. We all have right within us an endless supply of power from the same basic cosmic substance that all heavenly bodies and divine phenomena are composed of. This book was written with the intention of empowering those individuals who have been associated with lack, limited resources, and other low vibrational terms commonly linked to people living in the so called *hood* or predominately black and brown communities. These are actually the people endowed with the most potential for greatness and the ability to harness the previously mentioned vast and limitless nature of the universe. From this point on you would benefit greatly from disregarding any self limiting thought forms and tuning into the priceless and godlike forces waiting to be used right inside of you. This would not just benefit you, the individual but the world around you and your loved ones as well.

"The mere looking at externals is a matter for clowns, but the intuition of internals is a secret which belongs to physicians."

-Paracelsus

Healthy Again?

In the title of this book the word *again* is used indicating that we were healthy and in alignment with the universe once before. This perspective was not given to us in our modern-day public-school systems and is not found in most collegiate institutions. This legendary history has been maintained by some societies throughout the world while others are left to put the pieces together from studying and using the higher regions of their mind. We must stay present though and not fall victim to the vibrations that come with complaining about the past up until now. The fact that we were not raised learning about our true identity is not enough to hold us down. All is happening in divine order and it cannot be any other way. Our powers and potential are being revealed to us daily so let us make it a point to release what does not work so that we have room to use all the solutions being shown to us in this day and age.

Once upon a time, people had an intimate relationship with nature and were not as separate and divided as the people we see today. The world that we were born into currently is fairly new to the history of the earth. *The original people of the planet earth used the stars for instructions in their daily affairs and had a sound understanding of their relationship with the rest of the universe.* People may have moved at different paces and not agreed on everything, but things were much more different than what we see today. In many places when children were born, they had the village to assist with their growth and development, and they learned how to become useful to the collective. Knowledge of self was encouraged so that one would understand how to conduct his or herself in life and with things outside of self. A beautiful relationship between man and nature can be seen on each continent if we look back far enough into its history and the way people lived prior to the world's recent colonization.

Keep in mind that America, as we know it today is only a couple hundred years old. Imagine what you would be capable of by simply learning about what was stripped from you and complimenting that with putting forth the time and energy necessary to reverse the damage done.

(The words heal, holy, and whole have the same etymological roots.)

Ch.2: Genesis and The Absolute

In the beginning there was nothing but pure potential. Countless beings and things have been manifested from this place that is antecedent to all that exist, yet it still remains to be just as beneficial to the universe as it was when the first atom was formed. Just as there are many different names for the creator of the universe in our religious systems, the same is true in the scientific community. We have been taught to fragment our learning instead of acknowledging the way that all things are connected. Everything that has ever existed and all things that have yet to be manifested exist inside of what we call infinity and while it is hard to fathom for some, ***infinity is present inside of all finite things.*** Any finite person, place, or thing that one can imagine is made up of infinitesimal particles that work together harmoniously to create more complex entities and things to offer greater levels of service to the cosmic collective. This truth has been a reality since the beginning of time and even before time became a concept.

Studying the following terms and fields of study will take you back to the beginning if you are willing to let go of the falsehood that has not served you up until this point (NEXT PAGE).

Alternate Names For The Creator of The Universe

Infinity

The Absolute

Eternity

The Source

The Eternal Present Moment

Dark Matter

Blackness

Mother God

Zero Point Energy

Nothingness

Inertia

Counter Space

Ether

Triple Black Darkness

Primal Material

The Waters of Nu

Ancestors

Ch.3: On The Ancestors

We are the projections of our ancestors in this moment and our ancestors are the projections of us into the past. This is a holographic universe and everything is made up of light as we will explain throughout the duration of this book. We are our own ancestors and their genetics exist in our DNA. Our cells are literally composed of them. The eternal now exists in the present moment, which is really all there is. Our perception and our learned fragmented thinking cause us to mentally separate the so-called future and past. Our ancestors were so intelligent that they were able to create mythologies in order to share common interpretations of cosmic mechanics. A knowledge of self and of the universe one lives in increases the possibility and potential for balance between the two.

Our true history and origins can be shown to us in the world's most ancient forms of mythology. Our ancestors were so advanced that they used these mythologies to teach and show our relationship with astronomy, metaphysics, and even physiology. The western world has watered many of them down to throw us off from our past levels of achievement. None of the ancient systems come fully intact nowadays. We are going to have to continue to look within ourselves to completely recall what we are capable of. Another method would be to put multiple findings together in order to get a grasp on the bigger picture. Most people don't realize that many Europeans were commissioned to teach falsehood in order to elude and hide the history of the original man and woman. In order to be accepted into different collegiate circles, many black scholars were also forced to bare witness to certain theories and teach these false claims amongst our people. If we were to collectively remember who and what we are, the world would literally change overnight.

Modern astrophysics has accumulated a vast collection of information about the universe. This information however is expressed in a very different way when compared to our ancestors. Astrophysicists tend to express their findings in a very abstract manner via statistics, values, ratings, measurements, calculations, etc. none of which are incorrect per say but the ancients expressed their findings in a more creative and cohesive manner. The so-called ignorant and not so developed ancients some how managed to identify the interconnectedness in the celestial activities. The same laws and truths that were revealed back then are being identified in today's times. The difference being that our ancestors honored and revered the one primal substance in our universe and its various forms as opposed to our modern day scientists continuously clashing with each other from their fragmented perspectives.

The ancients knew that we were beings of spirit, mind, and body. It was taught that man was apart of the earth and the universe in general. The well being of the human body is influenced by the universe around it and vice versa. We also have the ability to attune ourselves to the creative intelligence permeating through the universe. Modern research reveals that the stone monuments and carvings of prehistoric times are not from primitive barbarians as we have been taught but instead are scientific instruments from ancient advanced civilizations. It has also been shown that many churches, stone circles, villages, etc. were constructed in areas corresponding to specific positions of heavenly bodies and also significant astrological phenomena i.e. rare celestial events. The cosmos in some societies was equated to a giant computer intelligently ushering us in and out according to our individual performances in our past lives.

An excellent way to get a better understanding of our ancestors is to study ancient Africa. While ancient America can also be studied and learned from, we know that at one point in time, all of the continents were once held together as a single land mass and that the one named Africa today was the portion that humanity had its origin in. Africa has an affinity with the Earth's point of inertia. Even to this day, it is the only continent to exist on four hemispheres and is the source of the majority of the world's minerals and natural resources. True African consciousness is wholesome and it does not entertain the spirit of separation. Both nature and God are considered and respected when identifying ones family and ancestral roots. We are all seen and honored as significant parts of the whole and as vehicles for eternity to exist through. New born babies, children, adolescents, adults, elders, ancestors, the elements of the universe, the spirit underlying and connecting all things and the creator are all respected as meaningful and relevant. Our western educational systems only seem supreme to what our ancestors achieved because much of what was accomplished in the past has been covered up or communicated in the modern world as mere mythology.

The Greek word mythos originally referred to "historical accountings of ancient peoples", and was redefined in the Middle Ages by the Roman Church to mean "imaginative and fanciful tales." It's important to keep in mind that within our modern languages there remains only a glimpse of the original meaning, mostly because ancient languages were symbolic and we have been indoctrinated with literal translations.

Ch.4: On DNA

Notice the important role of DNA (deoxyribonucleic acid) and how 2-3% of that DNA is used to upload or project what we call know of as the physical body very similar to how our modern day televisions depend on the LCD screens for the viewers to watch. The other 97-98% of our DNA is ignorantly referred to as "junk DNA" or noncoding DNA. This alone shows the obliviousness of our modern day educational system and institutions but leaves us with an opportunity to discover the more dormant portions of our existence. It is common knowledge in scientific circles that "junk" or noncoding DNA can be switched on and off. Our DNA has even been shown in recent years to be luminescent when placed in the proper range of wavelengths to expose the glow. The neglected power hidden in us that will be mentioned throughout this book is intimately connected to our ancestors and pieces of them still continue on in us and as us via their genetic remains.

The DNA molecule and its protein partners in the threadlike chromosomes found in the cell nucleus, maintain the specific linear sequence of the genes in passing on their hereditary message
of species development. The double helix is said to be the best macroscopic picture of the microscopic nucleic acid structure of the cell genes.

Section 1 Summary

If there's one word to describe the first section of this work, it is **reconnection**. The original people of this planet, OUR ancestors, were connected to everything around them – nature, the moon, the stars, their emotions, other people, everything. Because of this, they were able to answer the questions that have stumped us thousands of years later. Our ancestors understood who we are. For us to begin the healing of ourselves, we will need to tap back into this knowledge to re-find our power. "Awareness" is the first step towards true optimum health.

One thing about black people in America, we've been separated from our true history. Many of us can only trace our history back to the invention of hip hop, or the civil rights era. The American school system has only wanted us to know about our 400+ years in bondage. Truth is, our people have done much more, and have contributed pretty much everything to humanity. We are more than ex-slaves. We are some real powerful, magical people. That's why nobody or nothing has been able to keep us down.

Our ancestors used personification to explain "everything." While different civilizations used different descriptors in their storytelling – Mayan stories used animals like Jaguars, while Egyptian stories included animals like black cats, they always described the same things – what, when, where, why, and how of everything. Our ancestors were deeply connected to each other and all that's around them. However, humanity began a long period of unraveling.

Over time, especially times after the initial fall of most of Africa's premier empires such as the Egyptians, our ancestor's knowledge, teachings, and methods fell under heavy scrutiny and attack. Most of the historical buildings and monuments located in Northern/Sub-Saharan Africa were destroyed by Europeans when they began "exploring" the continent. An example of scrutiny is the European Age of Enlightenment of the 17th and 18th centuries. Our ancestor's elaborate stories of creation, tools, rituals, and personified maps of nature, the cosmos, and the soul were laughed at, even deemed evil or as nothing more than superstition. These "new" thinkers attempted to throw away all this knowledge, and history. For a long time, we were disconnected. However, truth can only be buried for so long.

Of the vast amounts of knowledge our ancestors had, perhaps the greatest understanding they had about everything, and something we need to understand today, is we possess everything we need to create the reality we want. Everything we need is already in us. We just must tap into it. Also, we must know that there's still so much remaining of our time as knowers on this planet. So much was destroyed, but so much remains. We have so much to our disposal in this new age of technology. We have no excuses. It's time to tap in and reconnect.

You Are More Amazing
Than You Realize

Ch.5: Know Yourself

"Mental liberation requires that we locate ourselves on the time line and map of human history, that we name and define ourselves, and that we rectify the problem of the loss of knowledge of self. Wherein we are overwhelmed by other people's knowledge."

-Dr. Asa G. Hilliard

Your center is the opposite of all things.

We are used to the circumstances that we experience today but we are unfamiliar with why these things are happening. It is our responsibility to study these things and to do something about it so that we don't continue to hand over the burdens that we currently have to our future generations. If we seek out the origin of the word educate we will find that it means to bring out that which is already latent inside of you. Dr. Na'im Akbar however alters the language used and teaches that it is a vehicle for the transmission of consciousness. This is important to know because with this view, we can see how a proper or improper education can affect a people respectively. (See Carter G. Woodson's *Education of the Negro* and *Miseducation of the Negro*) If we continue to identify ourselves with what we have been taught then we will remain limited by those beliefs and the consequences that come with them but if we change what we have been accepting and take the time to seek out the truth of who we are then we can have awareness and access to the unlimited amounts of power that we innately possess. Understand that the power has never departed from us but our awareness of it plays a crucial role in our ability to make use of it. How can we expect to draw from our divinely bestowed powers if we continue to reach outside of self like we have been taught, for solutions to our problems? We are bypassing the body and our personalities here when discussing the real self. We get spooked and turn away from conversations when the word soul is used because of how we have been brainwashed when in actuality it is essential to all that we know about ourselves. To simplify things here look at it as a small portion of the creative substance responsible for all things in existence. It is not religious as taught in doctrines but it is scientific and realistic. Your soul or your "portion" is just as important and as amazing as any other. We may be in different stages of our development but you are a child of God nonetheless who his destined to become greater than anything you have imagined thus far. Your soul is spiritual in nature and not physical as the world you have become familiarized with. This should spark some interest for you and your personal studies outside of this book. To get a more thorough understanding of what the self entails, we also encourage you to take a look into the origin of humanity and civilization. Study nature and that which sustains you effortlessly and also study God thru the universe as we all live, move, and have our experiences within it. These are just our suggestions but by studying yourself in a substantive and holistic manner, you will begin to discover and remember who and what you are and this will allow for you to get so much more out of life. It is up to our generation to take what our ancestors have cultivated and shared thus far to the next level and it is up to the individual to cultivate his or her own consciousness and to develop spiritually as a soul inhabiting a body.

Learning is wonderful and can be of great benefit to ones mind but the most important learning is about things pertaining to self. Notice how in the western world the books are centered around European history and highlight the accomplishments of Europeans. While this is a good example of placing yourself at the center of your findings, there are still many differences between their example and you. The European teaches that the self is the specific person and that inside of each human resides the ego. While there is a partial truth to this, their understanding is quite different from the African or the original concept of self, which places you back at the primordial cosmic material that all things are derived from and shows that you are a multidimensional being operating on different planes of existence simultaneously. You are your ancestors on back to the original atom and you are the source of all your experiences and manifestations.

For a more well rounded understanding of who and what you are, we employ you to research and study the works and efforts of the following historians and teachers.

Recommended Authors and Lecturers

Dr. John Henry Clarke

Dr. Yoseph Ben Jochannan

Chancelor Williams

Cheikh Anta Diop

Runoko Rashidi

Kaba Kamene

Ivan Van Sertima

Theophile Obenga

W.E.B. DuBois

Fard Muhammad

Marcus Mosiah Garvey

Carter G. Woodson

Amos Wilson

Steve Cokely

Professor Kaba Hiawatha Kamene

Ch.6: True Self

We would like to differentiate between the true self and the self we perceive ourselves to be when we come into contact with other sentient beings or what we have been taught in this backwards society. The self that many people see themselves as when they speak to others or walk to places has a very important role and we don't want to confuse this distinction with degrading this part of the person. Instead we simply want to use wisdom to insure that we are respecting the purpose of these two "sides" of the self. On one hand we are infinite beings with limitless potential and on the other end we have the temporal vehicle that have known up to this point as the human body. We have an exclusive obligation to tend to our portion of the former and we are responsible for its development as we learn our cosmic lessons in these temporary "spacesuits".

Many people today are immersed in the phenomena of the physical world but tend to forget about what is allowing them to do so in the first place. We wake up in the morning, wash up, eat breakfast, go to our respective work places, etc. all while projecting our attention solely onto the world and forgetting about where it comes from and what it is here for. When we are young or introduced to certain religions, we hear phrases like "in the world but not of it" and then we disregard it as adults when we think we have life figured out. The world around us continuously changes but the true self is a universal constant. We can choose to disregard and ignore ourselves or we can learn how to love ourselves. For those interested in genuine healing, the later is essential for any real progress. Also it is important to note that the more we actively love ourselves, the more capable we are of loving on others.

When we become more loving and accepting of ourselves, we start to break loose from self-destructive thought patterns and actions. Too often we abandon ourselves in pursuit of happiness from outside sources when in actuality we have everything that we need right inside of us. Loving ourselves entails being honest enough to let things go that harm us or hinder us from reaching our full potential even if we like and enjoy those things. It looks like respecting who we are enough to dismiss anything that interferes with our peace. In actuality an entire book can be written on this subject alone but here we want to make it clear that the love of who one truly is comes first before any real advancements can be made concerning ones restoration or realization of wholeness.

The universe is composed of many parts but is ultimately one coherent system. Everything in it is interconnected and interdependent. Its nature is spiritual and unseen forces sustain it i.e. the driving force behind planets and stars or the innate power in us that allows for us to have biological happenings like breathing that occur without our conscious input. The universe is rhythmic and its parts are complimentary to each other. We in our apparent individual forms are merely extensions of the universe and its splendor. The universal energy that we are composed of is spiritual. It is the animating awareness in all living organisms. Put in scientific terms, spirit is the dielectric field, which makes the mind and all forms of magnetism and expression possible.

Individual Empowerment

The next time you notice that you're doubting yourself, consider how insignificant a single atom may "seem." Even though many new discoveries have been made in regards to nuclear physics, it is still considered a universal building block. Alone it may appear to be inanimate or even useless from the perspective of the average human being however when it is cooperating properly with others, it can play its role in the creation process and take part in the construction of molecules, cells, tissues, systems, a physical body and a plethora of other possibilities. Many times people see themselves as weak, irrelevant or not capable but the truth is that they like the single atoms are qualified and more than able to manifest countless types of manifestations. They simply need to learn to believe in themselves and to learn practical methods of anchoring down solutions to solve their apparent problems. Just one person alone can teach a classroom, construct a building, perform music or alter the norm for a society but when he or she is allowed to harmonize with others, they can all produce manifestations more amazing than their mind could previously fathom. Now think back for a moment and reflect on the amount of possibilities present when atoms begin to join forces and notice how planets, stars, plants, and animals cooperate to make grander forms of creation. For some reason humans allow for their egos to keep them separated and in constant competition instead of harmonizing to be used by God for greater works. This is an obvious problem but we are creatures of habit and if we use a discerning eye we can see that we are continuously being encouraged and programmed to do things that keep our attention and minds off of collective thinking and cooperative actions amongst other things. As soon as we alter the paradigm by uniting for the greater good of humanity, we will create a shift powerful enough to dismantle the social systems that have proven to be detrimental to us as both individuals and humanity in its entirety.

We as the original people have options and have been through a lot collectively for millions of years. These past few hundred years have exposed us to some of the greatest amounts of pressure that we have ever experienced. On one end we have the options of busting or submitting to those posing as oppressors. On the other end we come out as the best possible versions of ourselves and we maintain that new state of existence perpetually until the universe sees fit to set us up with another grand challenge.

Ch.7: Self Love

A person can think about loving his or her self but no alterations will be made unless some type of action takes place. If we were to ask the average person if he or she loves their self, they would say "definitely" or give some kind of answer with conviction. If we asked that same person to make a list of their usual activities and to honestly place these activities into two columns labeled "beneficial" or "detrimental" to self, the detrimental column would have twice as many entries as the column labeled beneficial. This goes to show that our thoughts and actions are not always in alignment and that we have a lot of room for improvement individually as well as collectively as a people.

Self love is a possibility for the man or woman who believes in their self enough to draw from the infinite potential waiting to be released daily. The only thing holding us back is our self limiting beliefs and the false narratives that we have been taught from birth. We give our power away when we rely on saviors outside of ourselves to solve our problems for us. We have absolutely everything that we need right inside of us and we only magnetize the elements and circumstances to us and around us according to what we create as a reality within us. We have neurons in our brain and sensory neurites in our hearts that reconfigure themselves according to how we manage our consciousness. The future is much brighter than our recent past and it will manifest as fast as we choose to shift and do the necessary work to bring it about. We've been wasting our vital energies on realities that don't serve us and the universe loves us absolutely too much to allow that to continue to happen. This is the time to get clear and to be intentional about what we wish to manifest on the world stage.

Ch.8: Purpose is Primary

Each and every one of us was born for a reason and we have an obligation to fulfill that void for the benefit of the universe as a whole. We can look at our individual purpose like a piece to a puzzle and when we are in alignment with why we were born in the first place and we are walking in our purpose it compliments and serves everyone and everything around us. If we all chose to do this then it could be liken to a completed puzzle and we all would be able to benefit from the combination of our efforts. Even if one were to manifest the absolute best that he or she could, it would be nothing in comparison to what we could all achieve together. The universe is a workshop and a vehicle for eternity and we are the way that much of the work gets done. We can also look at our purpose like a divine assignment or a cosmic job. When we are not walking in our purpose, the universe recognizes us being out of order and steers us in the proper direction by any means necessary. If we get too far off track however, we may find ourselves subject to diseased states in our physical body, experiencing social problems with the world around us, or even terminated if Mother Nature feels that we've gone too far. Whatever the case may be, it is all out of love and done with our best interest in mind. The average person may find that to be harsh but we forget that we are seeing things with our physical eyes and our egos most of the time instead of looking at the bigger picture and trusting that the universe always has our back. It is our purpose that reveals our role in relation to the rest of creation and our true place in the cosmos. *Our journey to better health is a personal one and should not be determined by the standards or expectations of those outside of self. We are all living with different purposes that do not require the same choices or outcomes.*

Part 2 Summary

The true process of healing can begin the moment you realize how unstoppable you are. I say "can" because awareness is only half of the battle. You must act on what you know. When you know better, you do better. That completes the process of healing.

Some things you should be aware of in this quest for better health is:

- Our Creator created Creators
- Whoever feeds you leads you
- You should be your primary doctor
- We are connected to everything around us

We are Gods on this planet. We possess the gift of creating whatever reality we wish. You do not have to live a life of illness. You have the power to create a life of abundance, happiness, and great health. It's up to you to determine that path.

Knowing you have the keys means you should never give your powers to anyone else. Nobody should be in control of what you eat, how you make a living, or how you should be healed. That is your job. I've seen Asa say it repeatedly on social media while promoting his health consultation business, "If you know you are not eating right, or you are not exercising your body or brain, please do not inquire about my services. It isn't my job to heal you. That's your job. I am here to aid you in the work you are already doing."

You are more amazing than you realize. Once you realize how amazing you are, there is no excuse you can come up with to stay unhealthy or low. Take this "re-found" power (The power was always there. You just needed to find it) and use it to shape yourself into what you need to be to live your purpose. A part of that path requires you to be healthy physically, mentally, and spiritually.

The Universe

Ch.9: Cosmic Mechanics

Cosmic Mechanics can be understood as the crux of field theory and a foundation for cosmology that allows for us to comprehend the nature and function of the universe in and around us. All things in existence have some attribute or route to manifestation that makes them distinct to everything else however they all must follow the blueprint that the universe operates off of.

The Conjugate Nature of The Universe

The creator has a conjugate nature where on the inside exist a realm of pure potential, causes and possibilities and on the outside exists the world of expressions, effects, and externalizations. Conjugation entails that at least two things are joined and in this case it is the masculine and feminine forces of the universe. One is not greater or more important than the other and they both have a unique way in which they interact with the absolute.

The magnetic toroid (doughnut shape) and the dielectric hyperboloid (hourglass shape) together form a *holos,* which means whole or total and is where we get the word hologram. Totality is comprised of both principle and attribute i.e. water and wet or light and illumination. One is what a thing is essentially and the other is what the thing does. Its description is only possible because of how it makes itself known to the rest of the universe. The dielectric field and magnetism are the same essentially. Magnetism however is produced when there is a loss of energy or inertia (undisturbed pure potential) from pressure mediation in counter space. This is the beginning of understanding that nothing escapes the all. Things can only be expressed temporarily as they must eventually make their way back to the source. The source or primal material is the continual state of nonbeing, which continues to manifest itself. All things return here when they are complete or when their purpose is fulfilled. *(study source materials on Anpu or Anubis in our ancient Egyptian/Kemetic mythology and also centripetal convergence in modern day field theory.)*

All things in this book will be easier to understand once this simple concept is grasped.

Ch.10: On Dielectricity

A scientist by the name of William Whewell first coined the term dielectricity in response to a request from Michael Farraday who is known as one of the most influential scientist in the modern world. Dielectricity refers to the field in existence behind magnetism that can house and express its powers without the aid of a conductor. It exists in counter space and when there is any type of disturbance or perturbation there, it results in magnetism. Our ancestors were already familiar with this feature of the universe and revered it as the god Ausar. His counterpart and sister wife was worshipped as the Goddess Auset as she was responsible for the magnetism that made all of his potentiality possible. The dielectric field is shaped like a hyperboloid or an hourglass and is the inverse of the toroidal shape of the magnetic field it produces. Together they create a perfect sphere or the shape of totality.

Dielectricity is the fundamental field modality in our universe. Pressure mediation is what causes it to change in the same manner that temperature causes water to be altered from a vapor into a liquid or from a liquid into ice or structured water. As a result of this, everything in our universe works off of pressure mediation as the ether always takes the path of least resistance. An easy way to understand this is to think about the water going down a drain when the plug is removed or picture a latex glove filled with water and watch as the water moves in response to whichever way the glove is squeezed. It is also important to note here that dielectricity is not quantifiable as it is the prerequisite for all things that can be counted or measured. It is the cosmic substance that physicists are truly referring to when they speak of anything "quantum". While it is a scientific term, one can associate it with the spirit mentioned in mysticism or religious doctrines.

"Whenever the dielectric field "loses" energy it manifests spatially via magnetism."

-Ken Wheeler

Ch.11: On Magnetism

There is nothing in the universe that does not have an attribute. Otherwise it could not be known or described. The magnetic field underlying things is the reason that they appear or function the way they do. The magnetic fields are a direct result of the pressure that caused the loss of inertia or disturbance in the ethers, which preceded them. When the mind is poised and relaxed we are able to witness and pull from the power antecedent to all things. When we produce a thought however, a divergence occurs disturbing this peaceful state resulting in magnetism seemingly wielding the primal substance into the form of the thought. The magnetic field is made up of the same substance that it was derived from (dielectricity) and draws to itself the elements in the universe necessary for manifestation. Even the movements we make physically are magnetic in nature. In most situations, attention is needed to sustain the shape and endurance of the magnetic field. Negation allows for the convergence of the magnetic field back into the dielectricity or pure potential it came from. Peace then can be understood as our original state of existence both in the mind and externally in society.

Natural observations with magnets have led scientists to conclude that magnetism polarity is a property of ether. Previously they had been teaching that magnetism was a property owned by stones and certain materials. Our body's magnetic field pulls from the ether in and around us and allows for us to tap into unlimited amounts of energy and cellular potential. The plasma of the ether flows through our bodies effortlessly and is the very fundamental energy that animates the universe. All magnetic fields are shaped in the form of a torus or a doughnut, which is the inverse of the hyperboloid. At the center of every torus there is a black hole or point of inertia that remains undifferentiated. Both human beings and planets have torus foundations. Our greatest toroidal or magnetic field is found at the heart where we have the greatest concentration of mitochondria.

(Dielectric and magnetic lines of force cross at ninety degrees or right angles to produce light.)

..And God said, "Let there be light!"

Ch.12: On Light

Light denotes the presence of magnetism..

Wherever we are able to witness light, magnetism is present. Light as we know it is a byproduct of both dielectricity and magnetism. Our ancestors referred to this feature of the universe as Ra and in other cases, Heru, which is the prerequisite for the modern words hero, horizon, and hour. Heru was depicted as the son of Ausar in the same way that light can be understood as the son or child of dielectricity and magnetism as it is essentially the same in nature. Light can also be seen as a resurrected form of the dielectric field, which exists in counter space in the same manner that Ausar is depicted as living and ruling in the underworld. Volumes have been written on the subject of light but at this portion of the book we will simply use older linguistic terms to serve us in our endeavor to explain just a few ways that light is relevant to us.

Lumen is a Latin word for light and refers not to the light we see visibly but to the radiation, which passes thru the universe. Lumen is invisible but just as real as our consciousness. It refers to the condition of light transmitted by our sun and other stars. It is external to us until our melanin converts it into a more bioavailable form.

Lux **(Magnetism)** is also a Latin word for light but refers to the internal light, which is caused in our brain and mind. Lumen penetrates thru our personal atmosphere directly into our eyes and activates nerve cells as it is transformed back into Lux. This version of light that we are referring to as lux can be thought of as a psychic form of light created by our very own consciousness.

Nux **(Dielectricity)** is a Latin word for seed or kernel and refers to the inner core of our being in which the cosmic plan is constantly unfolding. Most of us are not familiar with this version of light because it is the dark unconscious portion where our primal drive springs from. It is symbolized by the black apparent emptiness of space because it is pure and unadulterated by thoughts, images, and sensations. It is the foundation of our being just as silence is the foundation from which all vibrations of sound result from. The basic field of consciousness is like an ocean and is so transparent and still that any disturbance or vibration in it or thru it will result in waves. These waves are the vibrations of the universe around us i.e. our sun, other stars, the sky, trees, crystals, people, etc. Everything we know of or can perceive is a disturbance, alternation or wavering in our nux.

Dielectricity, and meanings

Dielectricity	Spirit	First	Cosmic Clay	Primal Substance
Magnetism	Mind	Next	Workplace	Medium
Light	Body	Follows	Repository	Universe

Light as it manifests as the form we refer to as a photon is infinite. Photons are weightless and travel at maximum acceleration continuously until they are eventually changed into matter.

**The human body runs on light.*

Ch.13: On Fields

All manifested things have a field from which they are derived. A field can be defined as an ether perturbation modality, which is essentially a disturbance in the ether. Although we might conceive of there being different types of fields, there is ultimately one field, which all things exist in. Depending on the nature of a thing, it is manifested in a different place and proximity to others within the one major field according to its purpose and vibration. It is important to remember that all magnetism is made possible because of the potential latent within the dielectric field behind it.

In the scientific community, this has been differentiated into three interrelated aspects that affect the overall wellbeing of a sentient being.

Differentiated Levels of One's Personal Field	
L-Field	The portion where one's life force energy is housed and drawn from
T-Field	The portion where thinking happens and arrangement of the force occurs
M-Field	The portion where materialization takes place as a result of mental activity

(L-Field=Dielectricity)

(T-Field=Magnetism)

(M-Field=Condensed Light)

The human body's aura is produced by a derivative of the dielectric field, the L-field, given off due to the body's ability for superconduction. L-field harmony and emission come about as a result of having enough carbon in our cells. Carbon specifically emits a nerve force that enormously enhances our ability to deflect subnormal galvanometric energy. Relaxed and quiet, calm breathing has an outstanding effect on the blood.

Morphogenic Field

Our morphogenic field is a localized form of cosmic intelligence that reverts us to normal as quickly as possible. The fully assembled colloid structure is a result of a morphogenetic pattern instilled in the terrain of the substances that cause all characteristic life forms to materialize. A Morphogenic pattern is the intelligent blueprint field matter uses to assemble itself. An example of this is when the morphogenic field that creates a seed and holds all the information that the seed needs in order to develop into a plant or tree and the tree into plantations and forests.

Once a circle is created, as in the case of a morphogenic field, it becomes self-sustaining on the level of superconductivity, which is held in a delicate temperature range due to resonance. Our body's developed morphogenic field involves nerve junctions on both sides of the spine, which causes light to oscillate in and as us. Dipole fields arise from the brain's nerve structure and axons in the spinal cord. The oscillatory and diverging energies of a morphogenic field causes for minerals to assemble into the myriad of organic and inorganic structures. Our morphogenic field plays an unparalleled role in our healing processes.

Ch.14 Coherence

Coherency is when entities or substances are cooperating and functioning in a harmonious manner. Where coherence is found there is no room or tolerance for disturbances or opposition. An excellent analogy for understanding and being able to identify things that are coherent is to compare a five-watt light bulb to a five-watt laser. One is incoherent and radiates light in all directions which may be ideal for lighting up a room while the latter is concentrated and so intense that it can pierce and cut through dense materials. Black and brown people in urban areas and in the world's more neglected areas are typically unorganized and not in touch with each other. If we were to become coherent and laser-like in our communities, we could literally make major changes overnight. Because we are light beings, we have the capacity to function and manifest in the same manner as high powered machines that wield and alter the conditions of light.

Organization can even be understood as a form of spirituality. Coherency allows for us to add to one another's powers and potential in the same manner that cells ultimately form a human body. Atoms coagulate to develop molecules and molecules combine to form our cells and so on but when we can to the human level our egos give the illusion of separation when in actuality they should only be making us aware of our realm of influence and responsibility. When we learn how to transcend the apparent limitations of the ego Mother Nature will be able to express herself through us without obstruction. Coherency then can be viewed as a superpower in black and brown communities by enhancing both the individuals and the people involved collectively.

We have the potential to become an aggregate operating as a single entity.

Ch.15: On the Cosmos

Cosmos is used to describe the universe and its orderly and harmonious nature. Pythagoras whose name is derived from the Egyptian deities Ptah and Horus even used it all the way back in the so called 6th century B.C. Using the word cosmos as opposed to universe implies seeing it as a cohesive system or a grand entity. It suggests viewing existence as a holistic experience where all things live, move, and have their being in an identifiable oneness.

Cosmic dust is said to have its origin in stars and realities that existed far before our time. It is composed of various elements like carbon, oxygen, iron, and other atoms heavier than hydrogen and helium. These cosmic dust particles can remain suspended in space for long periods of time or make their way down to planets like Earth after entering areas with a strong enough gravitational pull. Thousands of tons of cosmic dust are expected to reach our planet's surface every year. Since it has been discovered by modern science, cosmic dust has helped to reveal information about phenomena like star formation and the development of solar systems. It also assists us in understanding the universe's recycling processes. Cosmic dust can be formed in stars and pulled away from other magnetic fields or disbursed out into space from star explosions. The dust then makes its way into the clouds of gases between other stars and is used for when the next generation of stars begin to form.

Presolar grains also known, as **stardust** is another term used to describe the residue left from supernovas. We have stardust in us as old as the universe. This means that our physical bodies are made of remnants of stars and powerful explosions that preceded us. Every man or woman can be understood as a local modern day star in and of themselves. We have a lot to remember post the world's most recent colonization by Europeans and their hidden helpers. Each and every one of us has the power and potential to make our lives revolve around us in the same manner that the sun magnetizes and wields planets around it. We are not just composed of stardust. We posses the history and forces embedded within them as well. In today's scientific terminology, the word colloid is used to describe these stardust particles in a more modern way.

Colloid can be used to describe a vast a mount of substances but it is usually mentioned to explain the presence of particles existing inside of another solution or medium. When the term colloid is used throughout the duration of this book we are referring to this phenomena in our physical bodies. Colloids responsible for the composition of our body are also synonymous with stardust as it makes itself known in us after combining and compression. Colloids or internal stardust can refer to microorganisms and cells that are assembled from minerals that retain and pick up cosmic energy from their constant spin orientations or what is insinuated by the Brownian movement. Colloids resist the pull of gravity, unless they are weighted down by moisture. They are substances consisting of ultra-fine particles suspended in a medium, like an insoluble mineral suspended in water. They are extremely small, typically measuring out to 0.01 to 0.001 microns in diameter. They are imperishable and at the end of human life, they are returned to the earth to exist in and as the soil where they can survive for millions of years until they are needed to participate in the livelihood of another sentient being. Colloids are the building blocks of DNA and have insoluble, heterogeneous, and multiphasic properties. Refer back to this knowledge whenever you forget about how ancient you truly are.

Colloidal Properties	
Insoluble	Incapable of being dissolved or broken down any further
Heterogeneous	Permitting different outcomes for chemical activities
Multiphasic	Having one or more phase or component

(We will use the term colloidal often throughout this book to refer to particles, minerals constituents, etc. as they serve as a bridge to tie us back to the universe around us.)

Hydrogen makes up over ninety percent of all the atoms in our universe. It is the only known element that can exist without neutrons. Hydrogen is said to have been discovered by the English scientist Henry Cavendish back in 1766 however our ancestor were very familiar with this basic element and referred to it as the deity Atum. At one point in time Atum was depicted as the god above all other gods because he was found to be present in all of them. All of the known elements in the universe are simply different combinations and arrangements of hydrogen. It is described as being colorless, tasteless, and odorless just as the blackness that it is an expression of. It is found mostly in stars and giant planets made of gas. Deep inside of stars, the pressure is so intense that hydrogen atoms are converted into helium atoms. This process is called fusion. In the same way that water can appear in 4 different phases, hydrogen can combine with different elements and change forms as well.

3 Types of Hydrogen	
Protium (H1)	No neutron and one proton (light hydrogen)
Deuterium (H2)	One neutron, one proton and one electron (heavy hydrogen)
Tritium (H3)	Two neutrons, one proton, and one electron (heavy heavy hydrogen)

The north (-) end of a magnet spins blood counterclockwise (left), decreasing hydrogen ions whereas the south (+) end causes blood cells to spin clockwise (right), increasing hydrogen production. The control of the hydrogen ion is an important reaction that takes place in the body. Spare hydrogen ions keep us looking and feeling youthful.

Ch.16: Star Formation

Hydrogen is mainly found to be in its H2 or Deuterium form when stars are produced. As alluded to previously, stars form as a result of hydrogen gases and cosmic dust accumulating and collapsing due to dielectric attraction or what we refer to as gravity. After the hydrogen in the star's core is exhausted, the star can fuse helium to form progressively heavier elements like carbon and oxygen until iron is formed. Up to this point, the fusion process releases energy. Iron is the most magnetic element in our universe and is not only found at the core of stars but also at the core of our blood in the compound known as "heme". While we are developed in our mother's womb over a period of approximately nine months, stars on the other hand take millions of years to develop from the time the initial gas starts to collapse up until the star is formed and begins to shine like a sun. The remaining cosmic particles or dust are used to create planets and other stellar objects that remain within the stars gravitational pull. The space in between stars is referred to as the interstellar medium. It is important to note here that most stars are not formed in isolation but as part of a group of stars or clusters. We here on Earth are also born into families and communities in order to offer greater services to the universe as a collective. The word star is found at the beginning of the word "start" which we use when we want to initiate and commence something. We must remember that we are able to do this because of the unlimited supply of fuel hidden inside of us, which not only parallels the power we see in the stars up above us but has its origin in the same universal force.

Astrocyte comes from the Greek words "64ender" meaning star and "kutros" meaning cell. These star cells are found in both the human brain and spinal cord and are collectively refereed to as *astroglia* due to their shape and potential. Just as the stars are plentiful in our universe, astrocytes are the most numerous cell type in our brains. They perform many different functions including the support of endothelial cells which form the blood brain barrier, maintenance of extracellular ion balance, regulation of cerebral blood flow, and they even have a role in brain cell regeneration.

Radiation from stars excites molecules of the air and ionizes the surrounding areas. It also penetrates the fluids of the human body. Humans, stars, and plants are all doing the same thing on different levels of manifestation. The light induction of chlorophyll in plants is only the first step in a long chain of events. In plants the light cycles produce oxygen and carbohydrates but in us the ATP created from various forms of secondhand light produces consciousness of the body. Consciousness is maintained in our sensory mechanisms by the continuous release of energy within the cell and nervous system.

Stars and planets are grouped into classes of magnitude according to brightness. Each said class is 2.512 times as bright as the preceding stellar body. The higher the magnitude the fainter the star seems to appear. Stars up to approximately magnitude 6.0 are visible to the naked eye.

Section 3 Summary

Here is a list of books that dive deeper into these concepts, as well as other concepts which will come up later in this book:

- *The Kyballion* by The Three Initiates (1908)
- *Powerful Planets Astrologically Considered* by Llewellyn George (1931)
- *Raja Yoga or Mental Development: A Series of Lessons* by Yogi Ramacharaka (1934)
- *Health and Light: The Extraordinary Study that shows how light affects your health and emotional well-being* by John N. Ott (2000)
- *Earth, Air, Fire, and Water: More Techniques of Natural Magic* by Scott Cunningham (2002)
- *Teaming with Microbes: The Organic Gardener's Guide to the Soil Food Web* by Jeff Lowenfels and Wayne Lewis (2010)
- *Vibration Law of Life* by W.H. Williams (2010)
- *Sea Vegetables, Harvesting Guide* by Evelyn McConnaughey (2012)
- *Minerals for the Genetic Code* by Charles Walters (2013)
- *Entheogens, Myths, and Human Consciousness* by Carl A. P. Ruck and Mark Alwin Hoffman (2013)
- *Soil Science Simplified* by Donald P. Franzmeier, William W. McFee, and John G. Graveel (2016)

- *Radical Regenerative Gardening and Farming: Biodynamic Principles and Perspectives* by Frank Holzman (2018)
- *Chasing the Sun: How the Science of Sunlight Shapes Our Bodies and Mind* by Linda Geddes (2019)
- *Pigments from Microalgae Handbook* by Eduardo Jacob-Lopez, Maria Isabel Queiroz, and Leila Queiroz Zepka (2020)
- *The Hormone Balance Bible: A Holistic Plan to Create Lifelong Health* by Shawn Tassone MD, PhD (2021)

The Sciences

Ch.17: Astronomy and Astrology

Astronomy is the oldest of the natural sciences. It is the prerequisite for what we know today as astrology.

In his book *The Culture of Astronomy*, Thomas Dietrick mentions that cosmic law informs natural law. Our ancestors also made it clear that the heavens were a divine expression and that it was also a means for communication between humanity and the creator. They expressed that the human body was created in the image and likeness of God and that it possessed divine characteristics. Since the ancients corresponded the human body with the cosmos, we find in different mythologies that they used for example what we refer to as Aries today to describe the head of the cosmic body and so on as we make our way from there throughout the remainder of the zodiac ending at the feet corresponding with Pisces. We on the other hand being unaware of our astronomical connections limit ourselves by not taking heed to some of the finest sets of instructions in existence. Many religious practitioners point upwards to the sky while speaking about God but are taught by their pastors or religious leaders that the worship or acknowledgement of stars is blasphemy or evil. This is pure ignorance and will be proven incorrect as the world's state of consciousness rises by the generation.

The stars and planets are a reflection and an expression of that which is eternal and we are here on earth to remember and assume our divine role in the absolute. All stars have their eccentric natures, properties, and conditions and make themselves known in us, the animals, the plants, and all other natural things. Everything that you can fathom has its character pressed upon it by the stars or planets responsible for its particular contribution to the universe. These characters contain and retain the specific natures, virtues, and roots, of their influencing stars/or planets and produce corresponding effects and operations.

Eleanor Kirk, in *The Influence of the Zodiac Upon Human Life*, wrote, *"There is a mind more interior than the animal mind...quickened by the solar fluids or planetary action, for it is the genius of the natural man. And there is still more interior mind, the spiritual, which is absolute over all earthly or planetary conditions, which glows and continues to ripen the divine human into celestial man...The stars may influence us, but God rules the stars, and when man recognizes God in himself, he can be dominated no longer by anything apart from God."*

Many ancient texts were also based on astronomical observations having to do with the movement of light. Karl Anderson, author of *Astrology of the Old Testament* or the Lost World Regained, gives insight into this idea. He explains that Genesis is derived from Gen-Isis (Isis being the Egyptian moon goddess) and makes many correlations between astronomical phenomena and characters in a variety of ancient texts. He writes,

"In the beginning God said, 'Let there be light: and there was light.' Light first springs from the first point in which the sun ascends at daybreak, or the life of nature commences in the point Aries... When God says 'Let us make man in our image,' "us" refers to the luminaries Osiris (sun) and Isis (moon)- the positive and negative principles, respectively. Osiris, as the sun is the life giver, and Isis, as the moon, is the producer. One represents spirit (sun as the principle form of light) and the other; matter (moon as light reflected in the darkness).

Egyptologist, John West, author of *Serpent in the Sky*, writes, *"Egyptian science, medicine, mathematics and astronomy, were all of an exponentially higher order of refinement and sophistication that modern scholars will acknowledge. The whole of Egyptian civilization was based upon a complete and precise understanding of universal laws. And this profound understanding manifested itself in a consistent, coherent and inter-related system that fused science, art, and religion into a single organic Unity...exactly the opposite of what we find in the world today."*

J. H. Hill in his book Astral Worship wrote the following, *"..religion having been based upon the worship of personified nature, it is evident that its founders fabricated its dogmatic element from their conceptions of her destructive and productive processes as manifested in the rotation and diversity of the seasons."*

Astronomical observations indicate inherent order and regularity in the motion of the planetary bodies. Our ancestors with their profound understanding of the cosmos referred to this regularity as *"the music of the spheres."* Many historians, including some Egyptologists claim that Egypt/Kemet did not have a refined system of astrology but when we continue to dig and seek out facts, we find that the opposite is true. Greek civilization is praised in many parts of the world and especially so in the west by European institutions but the first two Greek philosophers to attain astronomical and astrological knowledge (Thales in the 7th century BCE and Eudoxus in the 4th century BCE) both learned directly from their teachers in Egypt/Kemet.

Astronomy is the detecting and viewing of stars through different types of telescopes. Our eyes are our own personal telescopes and some individuals have vision so fine that they do not need the aid of external ones to assist them with viewing stars while others use intuitive means to accomplish this task i.e. the Dogon tribe of Mali in Northern Africa. The basis of this observational science is the grouping of stars into identifiable clusters called constellations. Astrology on the other hand is the science of corresponding celestial cycles with terrestrial events. Ancient astronomers used the constellations to determine the cardinal directions of the Earth, to measure the lengths of planetary movements, and to establish orientation of our planet within the universe. The groups of stars called constellations are typically named after mythical creatures (i.e. Orion and Sirius), objects (i.e. the Big Dipper and the Little Dipper), and animals (i.e. Leo and the Great Bear). They are a creative way to map and organize the celestial sphere. The celestial sphere can be described as the outer rondure of the heavens from the perspective of the Earth.

Section 4 Summary

For the longest time, humans have operated as though we've been lost or "low." That's because our planet goes through cycles where either the world's mass consciousness is either high and the humanity is in a good place, or mass consciousness levels are low and humanity is doing what it's been doing in modern times - abusing the planet, overusing its natural resources, and continuing to conflict amongst each other. Basically, we've been sleep because the planet is sleep. Thing is, our ancestors were aware of this because of their advanced knowledge of time, energy, and consciousness. Do some research on the Mayan civilization and their calendar system. They had a more accurate measure of time than we do today which helped them prophesize good or bad times.

Currently, the cycle is changing. We are waking up and our collective consciousness levels are rising. We are more aware. It's only up from here. Getting yourself together now presents the best chances of exploring and feeling the beauty of the whole. Yes, eating right and exercising is a part of that path, but understanding the universe, what to study about it, when to study it, where to look, and how to look at it is just as important. The next few sections dive deeper into the cosmic side of becoming a healthier being.

The Studies

Ch.18: On Star Clusters and Constellations

There are two general types of stellar assemblages or congregations. A star cluster is held together by dielectric attraction or what modern day science refers to as the gravitational pull from its members. The two types of star assemblies are called open clusters and globular clusters. Open clusters which were formerly called galactic cluster contain anywhere from a dozen to hundreds of stars, that are usually in an unsymmetrical or apparently random arrangement. Globular clusters on the other hand are older systems containing thousands to hundreds of thousands of stars closely packed in a symmetrical, roughly spherical shape. The *Pleiades* and *Hyades* are examples of open clusters and they can both be found in the Taurus constellation. The *Praesepe* also known as, the Beehive, containing about one thousand stars is another example and can be found in the Cancer constellation.

The first record of a globular cluster according to modern astronomers was Messier 22 in the Sagittarius constellation back in 1665. The next was Omega Centauri, which is visible to the naked eye and is located in the constellation Hercules. It is said to have been identified in 1677 after the invention of the telescope however since then an astronomical observatory was uncovered in Kenya dating back to so called 300 B.C. and

Galileo was also recorded mentioning that the ancients were familiar with telescopes. There are several societies like the Bambara, the Bozo, and the Minianka tribes in Africa who have proven to be just as familiar with the stars as the Dogon tribe in Mali from wisdom that has served their people for thousands of years.

Constellations, their locations, and their meanings

Constellation	Location	Meaning	Star Contained	Continued
Aries	N. Hemisphere	Ram	Shedar	Dat Al Cursa
Taurus	N. Hemisphere	Bull	Rigel	Bellatrix
Gemini	N. Hemisphere	Twins	Castor	Pollux
Cancer	N. Hemisphere	Crab	Al Tarf	Meleph
Leo	N. Hemisphere	Lion	Regulus	Algorab
Virgo	S. Hemisphere	Virgin	Spica	Beta Virginis
Libra	S. Hemisphere	Scales	Methuselah	Alpha Librae
Scorpius	S. Hemisphere	Scorpion	Antares	Shaula
Sagittarius	S. Hemisphere	The Archer	Kaus Australis	Terebellum
Capricornus	S. Hemisphere	Goat	Algedi	Nashira
Aquarius	S. Hemisphere	Water Bearer	Sadalsuud	Sadalmelik
Pisces	N. Hemisphere	Fish (Plural)	Alpherg	Parumleo

Aries

Aries is located in the first quadrant of the northern hemisphere (NQ1) and can be seen at latitudes between +90 degrees and -60 degrees. The Sun enters the sign associated with this constellation around March 21st each year signaling the beginning of a true new year. Aries is not just associated with the Ram via symbolism. It is known as an orientation sign and denotes the beginning of right ascension (RA) or the oriental first Right Ascension Midheaven (RAM). People born during this time should avoid taking too many stimulants. It would be wise of them to consume fruits and vegetables that support brain health. Herbs associated with Aries are mustard, eyebright, bay, and those with a pungent nature.

Taurus

Taurus is located in the first quadrant of the northern hemisphere (NQ1) and can be seen at latitudes between +90 degrees and -65 degrees. The Sun enters the sign associated with this constellation around April 20th each year. Those born during this time have great energy reserves, endurance, and stability. It would be wise of them to consume fruits and vegetables that support endocrine glandular functions and hormonal balance. Herbs associated Taurus are ground ivy, deadly nightshade, and vervain.

Gemini

Gemini is located in the second quadrant of the northern hemisphere (NQ2) and can be seen at latitudes between +90 degrees and -60 degrees. The Sun enters the sign associated with this constellation around May 21st each year. Those born during this time are known to have a keen mentality but can sometimes be indecisive. It would be wise of them to consume fruits and vegetables that support health lungs. Herbs associated with Gemini are lily of the valley, parsley, caraway, and lavender.

Cancer

Cancer is located in the second quadrant of the northern hemisphere (NQ2) and can be seen at latitudes between +90 degrees and -60 degrees. The Sun enters the sign associated with this constellation around June 21st each year and reaches its highest point or northern declination while in this zodiacal region. Those born during this time are known to be receptive, transforming, and nurturing but sometimes lacking in vitality. It would be wise for them to consume fruits and vegetables that cleanse and structure the lymphatic system. Herbs associated with Cancer are waterlily, chickweed, lettuce, and honeysuckle.

Leo

Leo is located in the second quadrant of the northern hemisphere (NQ2) and can be seen at latitudes between +90 degrees and -65 degrees. The Sun enters the sign associated with this constellation around July 22nd each year. Those born during this time are known to be dramatic and energetic but if the person is not spiritually developed or mature enough they can tend to be destructive. It would be wise of them to consume fruits and vegetables that nourish the heart and promote a healthy flow for the circulatory system. Herbs associated with Leo are wake robin, mistletoe, marigold, St. John's wort, and walnuts.

Virgo

Virgo is located in the third quadrant of the southern hemisphere (SQ3) and can be seen at latitudes between +80 degrees and -80 degrees. The Sun enters the sign associated with this constellation around August 23rd each year. Those born during this time are known to be hard workers and excellent servers but can tend to be people pleasers when they lack self-awareness. It would be wise of them to consume fruits and vegetables that cleanse the gastrointestinal tract. Herbs associated with Virgo are skullcap, fennel, mandrake, endive, and dill.

Libra

Libra is located in the third quadrant of the southern hemisphere (SQ3) and can be seen at latitudes between +65 degrees and -90 degrees. The Sun enters the sign associated with this constellation around September 23rd each year. Those born during this time are known to be balanced and great at managing relationships that they deem important. It would be wise of them to consume fruits and vegetables that nourish the kidneys and promote healthy elimination whether it be thru urination or defecation. Herbs associated with Libra are violet, pennyroyal, feverfew, catmint, burdock, and silverweed.

Scorpius

Scorpius is located in the third quadrant of the southern hemisphere (SQ3) and can be seen at latitudes between +40 degrees and -90 degrees. The Sun enters the sign associated with this constellation around October 23rd each year. Those born during this time are known to take things to the extreme whether it be in the bedroom or in the workplace. It would be wise of them to consume fruits and vegetables that promote healthy reproductive organs. Herbs associated with Scorpio are horehound, blackberry leaves, blessed thistle, leeks, horseradish, wormwood, and sarsaparilla.

Sagittarius

Sagittarius is located in the fourth quadrant of the southern hemisphere (SQ4) and can be seen at latitudes between +55 degrees and -90 degrees. The Sun enters the sign associated with this constellation around November 22nd each year. Those born during this time are known to be excellent teachers but can come across as condescending if they lack respect for someone. It would be wise for them to consume fruits and vegetables that strengthen the muscular system and promote elasticity for easy movement. Herbs associated with Sagittarius are agrimony, chicory, and red clover.

Capricornus

Capricornus is located in the fourth quadrant of the southern hemisphere (SQ4) and can be seen at latitudes between +60 degrees and -90 degrees. The Sun enters the sign associated with this constellation around December 22nd each year. Those born during this period are known to get better with time. It would be wise of them to consume fruits and vegetables that reinforce the skeletal system. Herbs associated with Capricorn are shepherd's purse, slippery elm, and knot grass.

Aquarius

Aquarius is located in the fourth quadrant of the southern hemisphere (SQ4) and can be seen at latitudes between +65 degrees and -90 degrees. The Sun enters the sign associated with this constellation around January 20th each year. Those born at this time are known to be unconventional and spontaneous. It would be wise of them to consume fruits and vegetables that naturally boost energy levels. Herbs associated with Aquarius are valerian root, lady's slipper, sage, and snakeroot, which is also known as spotted plantain.

Pisces

Pisces is located in the fist quadrant of the northern hemisphere (NQ1) and can be seen at latitudes between +90 degrees and -65 degrees. The Sun enters the sign associated with this constellation around February 19th each year. Those born during this time are known to be sensitive and inspirational. It would be wise of them to consume fruits and vegetables that promote healthy skin and pineal gland functioning. Herbs associated with Pisces are Irish moss, gentian, and ginger.

Ch.19: The Zodiac

The grouping of constellations on the celestial sphere that the ancient Egyptians paid special attention to became known as the "zodiac". The word zodiac means circle or animals or zoo disc. It is comprised of 12 constellations each of which is 30 degrees wide. The Egyptians/Kemetians used the zodiac as a tool to divide the ecliptic, which is the apparent path of the sun in the celestial sphere, into 12 equal zones equating to 360 degrees in total.

As the Earth, the sun, and the planets made their way thru the zodiac, the Egyptians/Kemetians were able to determine from which direction the energy of the universe flowed. They concluded that the direction from which a planet's energy flowed would give planetary energy a particular quality. Depending on which direction it was the energy would be either cardinal (initiating or catalyzing), fixed (fixed and static), or mutable (flexible and alterable).

Let us now look into astrology specifically, for a moment but not the watered down horoscope approach used by the mainstream astrologers today. Like most sciences practiced today, the true meaning of astrology has been kept away from the public so that the people would be more easily controlled and taken advantage of. To bypass that nonsense we can look to our ancestors for help. The first evidence of a zodiac is found at the temple of 86endera. The most famous as well as the most concentrated teachings can be found in ancient Egypt/KMT. Many of them are still in good condition today. This area is extremely dry and the ancients knew that dry conditions were excellent for preserving things. If it had not been for their efforts we would not have the understanding that we benefit from today.

From Aries to Virgo we see a focus on the perfection of the physical body and from Libra to Pisces we focus on the development of the spirit in that body.

Zodiac Signs Attributes

Zodiac Sign	Feature	Other	More
Aries	Assertiveness	Pressure	Impression
Taurus	Materialism	Substance	Receptivity
Gemini	Mentalism	Intelligence	Thinking
Cancer	Sentiment	Nurturing	Caution
Leo	Power	Expression	Ability
Virgo	Refinement	Perfection	Practice
Libra	Consideration	Harmonization	Relationships
Scorpio	Creativity	Transformation	Wielding
Sagittarius	Development	Elevation	Higher Mind
Capricorn	Reputation	Representation	Demonstration
Aquarius	Enlightenment	Humanitarianism	Inventiveness
Pisces	Preeminence	Polishing	Transcendence

Ch.20: On Planets

The Sun (Vitalize and Fuel)

The sun transits the 12 signs in approximately 1 year. It is associated with the cells, the human body in general, the heart and the circulatory system. The sun governs vitamin A, vitamin D, and PABA. It is responsible for the vitalizing principle in us and is the original manufacturer of the physical body. The Sun's house position indicates in part the individual's energy levels and resistance to disease. The Sun's sign location indicates the regions of the body that are most subject to malfunction and disease.

Mercury (Analyze and Interpret)

Mercury transits the 12 signs in approximately 1 year due to its close proximity and influence from the Sun. It is associated with the nervous system, speech organs, hearing organs, and health throughout one's youthful stage. Mercury governs vitamin B1 (also known as thiamin), the B complex in general, and thyroxin. It is responsible for our ability to communicate and think intelligently.

Venus (Exchange and Attract)

Venus transits the 12 signs in approximately 1 year. It is associated with our hormones, the glandular system, the kidneys, and the veins. Venus governs vitamin E and niacin. It also governs copper, molybdenum, and chromium. It is responsible for the beauty in things and our ability to exchange energy with others. Venus rules physical sensations and the female genitalia.

The Moon (Patience and Formation)

The moon transits the 12 signs in 27 days, 7 hours, and 43 minutes thus the "28 day moon cycle" we hear of when we learn about the waxing and waning phases. The moon governs B2 (also known as riboflavin). It also governs water fluorine and potassium. It is responsible for cycles and processes that require for us to have patience. It is associated with all bodily fluids, the lymphatic system, fertility, and our mucous membranes. The moon rules reflexes, acts that do not require conscious thought, and habit patterns.

Mars (Action and Penetration)

Mars transits the 12 signs in approximately 22 months. It is associated with the muscles, our sexual functions, and ones middle ages in life. Mars governs B12 and its contributing roles in making both DNA and blood. It also governs cobalt, iron, and phosphorus. Mars rules physical action and movement. It rules the red blood cells and adrenaline, which mobilizes the body's defenses when we are threatened from external sources. Mars is associated with the male principle and governs the external portion of the male genitalia i.e. the penis/phallus.

Jupiter (Reward and Expansion)

Jupiter transits the 12 signs in approximately 12 years. It is associated with the liver, organic systems, and some aspects of blood development. Jupiter governs vitamin B6 (also known as pyridoxine), vitamin K, choline, inositol, lecithin, and biotin. It also governs sulfur and selenium and their essential roles in bodily function. Jupiter has as its principle function the growth and expansion of the body.

Saturn (Parameters and Discipline)

Saturn transits the 12 signs in approximately 29½ years. It is associated with the skin, bones, teeth, hair, old age, and the hardening of tissues. Saturn governs Vitamin C and folic acid. It also governs calcium and its multiple roles in the body. Saturn has as its principle function forming the structure of the body and establishing limits. Saturn also highly influences the parathyroid glands in the neck, which regulate the metabolism of minerals necessary to bone formation.

Uranus (Originality and Impulse)

Uranus transits the 12 signs in approximately 84 years. It is associated with the body's pulsations, breathing patterns, peristalsis, and all functions that depend on rhythm. Uranus governs zinc. It highly influences the involuntary or autonomic nervous system, which controls involuntary functions of the body such as digestion, respiration, and heartbeat.

Neptune (Belief and Imagination)

Neptune transits the 12 signs in approximately 165 years. It is associated with bodily weakness, paralysis, the pineal gland, and the solar plexus. Neptune governs a B vitamin called pantothenic acid as well as all toxins, poisons, alcohol, and heavy metals. It rules the spinal fluids along with the moon and is associated with various extra sensory perception or ESP processes. It is classically called the "planet of deception" but essentially rules over what we believe and what we accept as truth.

Pluto (Birth, Death and Transmutation)

Pluto transits the 12 signs in approximately 248 years. It is associated with our capacity to regenerate and the rectum. Pluto governs enzymes and their activities in the body. It rules over abnormal cell growth like tumors, birthmarks, warts, and moles. It also associated with replicative processes thus the mentioning of enzymes, which catalyze chemical reactions within the cell, and the hereditary component involving DNA in the cell's nucleus.

Planets and their Characteristics

Planet	Feature	Other	More
Sun	Authority	Creativity	Vitality
Mercury	Communication	Calculation	Learning
Venus	Reciprocity	Harmony	Exchange
Earth	Embodiment	Personification	Plane of Inertia
Moon	Sensitivity	Emotion	Reflection
Mars	Dynamism	Enthusiasm	Potency
Jupiter	Expansive	Organizing	Advancement
Saturn	Contraction	Parameters	Protection
Uranus	Originality	Individuality	Exclusivity
Neptune	Imagination	Belief	Acceptance
Pluto	Birth	Destruction	Transmutation

Ch.21: On Astrology and Health

Like any other circle, the zodiac is divided into 360 degrees and each zodiacal sign is composed of 30 of those degrees resulting in 12 portions that also have anatomical and biological correspondences. The parts of the body ruled by those signs are as follows:

Aries: Head & Cerebrum, Initiatory

Taurus: Neck & Cerebellum, Stabilizing

Gemini: Lungs & Arms, Versatility

Cancer: Breast & Stomach, Tenacious

Leo: Heart & Spinal Column, Inspired

Virgo: Intestinal Tract, Industrious

Libra: Kidneys, Harmonious

Scorpio: Sex Organs & Rectum, Mystery

Sagittarius: Hips & Thighs, Expansive

Capricorn: Knees, Responsible

Aquarius: Calves & Ankles, Unconventional

Pisces: Feet, Transcendental

We often hear that the body is a universe and is one of the finest forms of technology in existence. It truly is and has its own resonations with the celestial canopy above us. When we look out at the stars at night we can rest assured that the mind-blowing phenomenon above us exists in us as well. The following is a modernized explanation of our affinity with these divinely placed stellar wonders. Notice how each of our body's systems has its own cosmic correspondence. The function of each system also resembles the way nature is expressed when the Sun is shining through a particular star cluster or what we would call a constellation. As opposed to anatomical associations to the signs starting from the top of the body and making their way to the bottom, the systems differ as they make their way from the innermost portions of the body to the outer.

The bodily systems ruled by the signs are as follows:

Aries: Nervous System

Taurus: Endocrine System

Gemini: Respiratory System

Cancer: Lymphatic System/Immune System

Leo: Circulatory System/Cardiovascular System

Virgo: Digestive System

Libra: Excretory system

Scorpio: Reproductive System

Sagittarius: Muscular System

Capricorn: Skeletal System

Aquarius: Meridian System

Pisces: Integumentary System/Skin

Ptolemy is credited with writing a book called the *Tetrabiblos,* which is what much of the modern taught astrology known to the public is based on. He was not aware of the functions of the organs in detail, which were rediscovered only recently. Our ancient African priests and medicine men however were knowledgeable in regards to our inner workings and they also had an understanding of life before and beyond what we know as the physical world. This wisdom was not exclusive to those who practiced the healing arts but was taught in many of our mystery schools as well as our villages and kingdoms that preserved our timeless history and spiritual astuteness.

The space we occupy, which is made up of the physical material that composes us has physical attributes that involves the rotating of electrons orbiting a mass of nucleons and positrons that are constantly being moved around inside of us. In turn, this movement is affect by the Earth and is pulled by the Sun, which orbits the galaxy in a perpetual motion. The inner world of our body is the microcosm that reflects the greater outer world around us, the macrocosm.

Ch.22: Systems of the Human Body

1st Portion misnamed Aries consists of the Central Nervous System, (Brain, Spinal Colom, and Neurons.)

The 1st portion's mineral composition is calcium, iodine, magnesium, manganese, phosphorus, potassium, silicone, sodium, and sulfur. The function of nervous system is to serve as a medium via nerves and neurons to transport and transform ideas and thinking into chemical and biological correspondences to be carried out by the body.

1st Portion Correspondences

1st Portion Correspondences	
Self Awareness	Cognizance
Singularity	Brain Health
Action and Sensory Coordination	Internal Light House
Coherence	Electrical Signaling

2nd Portion misnamed Taurus consists of the Endocrine System

(Pineal, Hypothalamus, Pituitary, Thyroid-Parathyroid, thymus, pancreas, Adrenals, Prostate, Uterus, Ovaries, and Testicles)

The 2nd portion's mineral composition is multifaceted due to its multi-gland configuration. The pineal gland is composed of manganese, phosphorus and sulfur. The hypothalamus is composed of chlorine, iodine, magnesium, potassium, and sodium. The pituitary is composed of iodine, manganese, phosphorus, and sulfur. The thyroid is composed of chlorine, iodine, magnesium, potassium and sodium. The pancreas is composed of chromium, manganese, and potassium. The prostate is composed of magnesium, silicone, and zinc. The testicles are composed of magnesium, manganese, phosphorus, silicone, and zinc. The vaginal canal is composed of sodium, potassium, magnesium, and calcium. The function of the endocrine system is to secrete chemical messengers called hormones directly into the bloodstream. The endocrine system also works with the nervous system to control and coordinate many bodily functions and maintain homeostasis.

2nd Portion Correspondences

2nd Portion Correspondences	
Alignment	World of Reflections
Goal Setting	Principles
Proper Selection	Value System
Prioritization	Emotional Fluctuations

3rd Portion misnamed Gemini consists of the Respiratory System,

(Lungs and Air Passage Ways.)

The 3rd portion's mineral composition is manganese, phosphorus, and silicone. The function of the 3rd portion is to provide oxygen to body's cells while removing carbon dioxide. This oxygen is taken from the lungs into the blood where the cells collect it in order to use for the oxidation of glucose (from fruit) for ATP production.

3rd Portion Correspondences

3rd Portion Correspondences	
Perception	Lung Health
Centering Self	DMT Production
Complete Breathing	Diaphragm Expansion

4th Portion misnamed Cancer consists of the Lymphatic/Immune System

(Lymph Nodes, Lymphatic Vessels, Immune Cells, and Water)

The 4th portion's mineral composition is mainly hydrogen and oxygen but more specifically H302 in a healthy body as structured water ensures the protection of hydrogen and the exclusion of toxic and unnatural substances. The function of the 4th portion is to drain, cleanse, and defend the body. The lymphatic System filters the bodily fluids.

4th Portion Correspondences

4th Portion Correspondences	
Behavior	Defense Systems
Culture	Military
Foundation	Habit Formation
Nurturing	Nourishment

5th Portion misnamed Leo consists of the Circulatory and Cardiovascular System/Blood System

Veins, Arteries, Capillaries, Heart, and Blood

The 5th portion's mineral composition is multifaceted as well. The blood is composed of calcium, copper, iron, potassium, sodium, and zinc.

The blood vessels are composed of magnesium, silicone, and sulfur. The heart is composed of calcium, iron, magnesium, phosphorus, and potassium. The function of the 5th portion is to transport nutrients from food, oxygen, waste products, hormones, and other substances that need to be relocated or removed.

5th Portion Correspondences

5th Portion Correspondences	
Discipline	Refinement
Self-Control	Circadian Rhythm
Creativity	Blood Flow
Blood Quality	Exercise

6th Portion misnamed Virgo consists of the Digestive/Alimentary Tract(Gastro Intestinal Tract)

Mouth, Esophagus, Stomach, Duodenum, Small Intestines, Large Intestines

The 6th portion's mineral composition is calcium, chlorine, iron, iodine, potassium, and sodium. The function of the 6th portion is to break down the foods we eat into substances the body can absorb and use for energy, repair, growth, and development. Nerves from every system of the body congregate here.

6th Portion Correspondences

6th Portion Correspondences	
Hard Work	Assimilation
Details	Equilibrium
Gut Health	Perfection
Microbiome	Analyzing

7th Portion misnamed Libra consists of The Excretory system

Kidneys, Bladder, Urethra

The 7th portion's mineral composition is in 2 places. The bladder is composed of fluorine and silicone. The kidneys are composed of calcium, chlorine, fluorine, iron, magnesium, and manganese. The function of the 7th portion is to filter the blood and excrete urea, excess water, and waste from the body.

7th Portion Correspondences

7th Portion Correspondences	
Self Reflection	Partnerships
Balance	Elimination of unnecessary substances
Win/Win Relationships	Liberation of Consciousness

8th Portion misnamed Scorpio consists of the Reproductive system

Prostate, Testicles, Penis and its Vessels, Smaller Organs, Uterus, Ovaries, and Fallopian Tubes

The 8th portions mineral composition varies in men and women. The prostate is composed of magnesium, silicone, and zinc. The testicles are composed of magnesium, manganese, phosphorus, silicone, and zinc. The function of the 8th portion varies in men and women.

In the male the function is to produce, maintain, and transport sperm and semen while in the female the function is to produce the female egg (ova or oocytes) necessary for reproduction. Both male and females reproductive systems are designed to ensure the continuation of the hue-man family. These systems also serve as a medium for regeneration and the reversal of age.

8th Portion Correspondences

8th Portion Correspondences	
Youthfulness	Shared Wealth & Prosperity
Restoration	Sexual Energy
Age Reversal	Transformation
Regeneration	Creative Energy

9th Portion misnamed Sagittarius consists of the Muscular system

Muscles, Tendons, and Ligaments

The 9th portion's mineral composition is calcium, chlorine, magnesium, manganese, potassium, phosphorus, and selenium. The function of the 9th portion is primarily for movement throughout the body. The muscles also serve as sensory organs.

9th Portion Correspondences

9th Portion Correspondences	
Progression	Fascia
Expansion	Measurement
Spiritual Development	Growth

All Natural Protein Builders

All Natural Protein Builders	
Fonio	Quinoa
Amaranth	Black rice
Walnuts	Wild Rice
Tahini	Pumpkin seeds
Sunflower Seeds	Bamboo
Chickpeas/Garbanzo Beans	Hemp Seeds
Kamut	Brazil Nuts

10th Portion misnamed Capricorn consists of the Skeletal system

Bones and Joints

The 10th portion's mineral composition is calcium, chromium, magnesium, phosphorus, and zinc. The function of the 10th portion is to serve as the body framework and structure for other bodily systems. Shape or form denotes how a cell or body part functions. The shape of our vocal cords determines our voices, the shape or arrangement of the light determines what we see, the shape and composition of matter determines how it feels, etc. The shape of a molecular structure is determined by repulsion. This is the push or force of a said material, which determines its distance and relationship or chemistry with the other minerals around it.

10th Portion Correspondences

10th Portion Correspondences	
Reputation	Crystallization
Organization	Quartz
Blueprint	Lifestyle
Mapping	DNA

11th Portion misnamed Aquarius consists of the Meridian system

Astrocyte Cells and Nerves

The 11th portion's mineral composition is copper, iron, and selenium. The function of the 11th portion is to regulate the energy of the body in order to maintain balance and proper energy distribution.

11th Portion Correspondences

11th Portion Correspondences	
Devotion	Massage Therapy
Teamwork	Daily Stretching
Acupuncture	Hatha Yoga

12th Portion misnamed Pisces consists of the Integumentary system

Skin and its 7 Layers

The 12th portion's mineral composition is copper, manganese, silicone, sodium, and sulfur. The function of the 12th portion is the internal and external worlds. It protects us from and allows us to feel the world outside of us. Our skin absorbs light and converts it into instructions for maintaining order throughout the rest of the body. For premium skin health, you should be able to consume the products that you put on your skin. They will more than likely be enjoyed better on your skin and not on your tongue but it should be noted here that everything put on the skin eventually makes its way down into the bloodstream. (An excellent example of this would be products at *www.bluelotusessentials.com*)

12th Portion Correspondences

12th Portion Correspondences	
Navigation	Adjusting
Undoing	Polishing
Believing	Acceptance

Excellent Skin Foods

Excellent Skin Foods	
Batana Oil	Marula Oil
Calendula Oil	Shea Butter
Hemp Oil	Cocoa Butter

What we refer to, as creation is nothing more than the differentiation or formation of the primal material of the universe. While the ego is responsible for the illusion of our mental and spiritual separation, the skin is responsible for our apparent physical separation as it gives the appearance of parameters and distinguishes between the inside and the outside of a person. We are all interconnected on many levels but the skin reminds us of what we are undeniably responsible for. What we term the skin is essentially a combination of minerals magnetically suspended and held together in water.

Additional Systems

Our *Endocannabinoid Receptor System* allows for us to commune with the special plant categorized as cannabis and also serves as a regulator of our immune responses, intercellular communication, appetite, metabolism, and a plethora of other bodily features.

Our *Sensory System* is a specialized portion of the nervous system that deserves its own attention and respect due to the fact that it gives us the ability to discern between our inner and outer worlds. Meditation can be used to enhance the capabilities of this system as it works to assist with our awareness of energies and substances.

Ch.23: Zodiac Pairs

The six pairs of the zodiac signs correspond to clearly established anatomical regions of the body as well as to the tissues and organs in those regions. Each pair also corresponds to some physiological process that is required for life. The signs and the planets in those signs form the blueprint for what is known as medical astrology. Following are the sign pairs and the anatomical regions that they rule over.

Aries and Libra:

Anatomically, Aries rules the skull, the brain, the upper row of teeth and everything in the superior portion of the head. Libra rules the kidneys and the organs involved with excretion. Physiologically, the function of this zodiacal pair is regulative. The kidneys maintain the salt and fluid balance of the body and keep toxic substances from building up to a dangerous level. The medulla oblongata contains the nerve centers that regulate heart and respiratory rate, while the brain general regulates most physical and mental activities.

Taurus and Scorpio:

Anatomically, Taurus rules the lower jaw and the throat region, which includes the larynx or voice box, the tonsils, upper cervical vertebrae, tongue, mouth, and thyroid gland. Scorpio rules over the reproductive organs, the rectum, and in men, the prostate gland. Physiologically, this zodiacal pair functions via consumption, elimination, and procreation. The solid matter from digestion passes through the Scorpio region, and the waste products of respiration i.e. water and carbon dioxide pass through the mouth in the Taurus region.

Gemini and Sagittarius:

Gemini rules the respiratory system, which includes the lungs, thoracic cavity, diaphragm, trachea, and the arms from the fingers to the shoulder blades. Sagittarius rules the hips and the upper portion of the legs on down to the knees, as well as the sciatic nerve. Physiologically, this zodiacal pair functions via distribution and locomotion. Gemini rules all of our body's tubes while Sagittarius rules over locomotion as it allows for us to move from one place to another.

Cancer and Capricorn:

Anatomically, Cancer rules the upper abdomen and the upper portion of the liver. It also rules all of our body's containers i.e. the breasts, the stomach, the womb, the peritoneum around the abdominal cavity, the pleural sac around the thoracic cavity, the pericardium surrounding the heart, and the meninges, which are the sacs surrounding the brain and the spinal canal. Capricorn rules over the knees and the entire skeletal system, which gives structure to the body. This zodiacal pair functions via protection and structure.

Leo and Aquarius:

Anatomically, Leo rules over the heart and the spinal vertebrae directly behind the heart. Aquarius rules over the lower portion of the legs. It also rules over the oxidative process, which energizes the body. Physiologically, this zodiacal pair functions via circulation and energizing. The heart, via the pumping of the blood, energizes and stimulates everything inside the body. This pair is also responsible for the basic chemical reaction that takes place in every cell of the body by way of oxidation, which is the combination of oxygen and glucose to produce energy.

Virgo and Pisces:

Anatomically, Virgo rules over the gastrointestinal tract while Pisces rules over the skin and the feet. Physiologically, this zodiacal pair functions via assimilation, discrimination, and isolation.

Typically when one area of the body is diseased or operated on, the anatomical region corresponding with the opposite sign is affected as well.

Tissue Cell Salts

While the zodiac corresponds and resonates with the systems of the body, it does the same on a smaller scale inside of the plasma of the blood. This particular correspondence is found in the tissue cell salts. There are 12 in total and each of them has a signature from a particular portion of the zodiacal belt. Tissue cell salts are known as inorganic minerals that do not contain carbon. Mineral components, plants, and animals that contain carbon are organic. The tissue cell salts are isolated components of our body's tissues. When our body is deficient of a specific cell salt it can be related to symptoms of an illness. To use the biochemical tissue salts as a remedy you must match your issues to the cell salt that serves as a solution to the said symptom(s). Western education teaches us that these inorganic minerals are the only substances that the cells in the body cannot reproduce by itself and that they must be taken either in a supplement or eaten in foods that contain them naturally. The authors are of the mind that this is only true for persons with bodies and minds that are not fully activated as some individuals have developed to the point that they can cause biological transmutation in order to create what they please.

The twelve tissue salts are typically taken in tablet form where the minerals are ground and triturated or turned into a fine powder. The minerals in the tablets are too low to have a detectable effect on the body's mineral and electrolyte levels. It is believed that this low level is what stimulates the cells to be restored back to their normal healthy state.

The Aries Cell Salt:

Potassium phosphate also known as "Kali Phos" is the Aries tissue cell salt. Its principle effect is on the nerve cells, especially the brain cells. It unites with a protein called albumin and also with oxygen to form the "gray matter" of the brain. It is used for healing and also as an antiseptic. It is required for cell growth and cell reproduction. Potassium phosphate is used to treat all forms of mental fatigue, depression, insomnia, hysteria and headache. Due to its antiseptic properties, it is reported to be effective in treating certain skin conditions, especially when there is irritation or burning involved. It helps to keep pores clean and can be effective in the treatment of problems with acne. Potassium phosphate is the most potent of all the cell salts. It should always be taken with iron phosphate, which we will discuss shortly.

(Potassium phosphate can be found in lettuce, cauliflower, olives, cucumbers, spinach, radishes, cabbage, onions, pumpkin, walnuts, and apples.)

The Taurus Cell Salt:

Sodium sulfate also known as "Nat Sulph" is the Taurus tissue cell salt. Its main function is the elimination of excess fluid from the body. Sodium sulfate has the property of chemically attracting large volumes of water.

It is known to be especially important in the digestive process for the production of bile and pancreatic fluids and also for proper kidney functioning. It is used for gallstones, kidney stones, jaundice and constipation. Sodium sulfate is also used to reduce swelling and other edematous conditions.

(Sodium sulfate can be found in beets, spinach, horseradish, cauliflower, cabbage, radish, cucumber, onion, and pumpkin.)

The Gemini Cell Salt:

Potassium chloride also known as "Kali Mur" is the Gemini tissue cell salt. It is important in the formation of most cells with the exception of bones and helps them to retain their shape. Potassium chloride enables the body to assimilate other nutritional substances from food, and an insufficiency of this salt has been known to result in unwanted weight loss and malnutrition. It is used with iron phosphate to relieve inflammation and irritation as well as in all respiratory problems like colds, hay fever or postnasal drip. Sore throat, tonsillitis, swollen glands and many childhood related diseases such as measles, chicken pox, and scarlet fever have been reported to be helped by the administration of potassium chloride. It has also been proven to be helpful in treating dry and scaling skin conditions like dandruff and psoriasis. When complimented by silica, it is shown to be helpful in reducing pitting after chicken pox, or acne, and helps reduces formation of scar tissue in burns.

(Potassium chloride can be found in asparagus, green beans, beets, sprouts, carrots, spinach, tomato, sweet celery, oranges, peaches, pineapples, apricots, pears, and plums.)

The Cancer Cell Salt:

Calcium fluoride also known as "Calc Fluor" is the Cancer tissue cell salt. It is a constituent of hard tissues like teeth, bones, fingernails, the lens of the eye, and also the elastic fibers in muscle tissue. When a person is deficient in calcium fluoride, the elasticity throughout their body is diminished and eventually lost if the problem worsens. The most obvious indicator of insufficient calcium fluoride is the appearance of open cracks or openings in the skin folds like in between fingers and toes, in the anus, the corners of the mouth and behind the ears. It has been proven to be effective in the treatment of hemorrhoids, varicose veins, receding gums, loose teeth, cataracts, blurred vision, bony lumps, the hardening of arteries and valvular heart disease. It is best if calcium fluoride is administered with silica as they compliment each other well when restoring the body. Some holistic doctors and homeopaths prescribe this salt for expecting mothers, as it is known to make abdominal tissues more supple for an easier delivery and to prevent sagging of the abdomen after the child is born. It also does the same for breasts after years of breast-feeding. Always be sure to seek the advice of a physician before using during a pregnancy.

(Calcium fluoride can be found in eggs, cabbage, lettuce, watercress, and pumpkin.)

The Leo Cell Salt:

Magnesium phosphate also known as "Mag Phos" is the Leo tissue cell salt. It is associated mainly with motor and sensory nerves that carry impulses to and from the brain. Due to the sensory nerves transmitting pain, it is often called the "anti-pain" salt and has been known to be effective in in relieving headaches and migraines. Magnesium phosphate has a soothing and relaxing effect on the body and has proven to relieve nervous tension. Insufficient amounts of magnesium can cause convulsions and muscular spasms. It has also been recorded in treating issues like nervous constipation. Magnesium phosphate, potassium phosphate, and ferrum (iron) phosphate can be taken in rotation for practically all forms of tiredness and exhaustion from overwork, insomnia, spasms, cramps, and neuralgia. If this regimen is used, most doctors prescribe potassium phosphate with meals, ferrum or iron phosphate after meals, and magnesium phosphate in the morning, afternoon, and again before sleeping at night.

(Magnesium phosphate can be found in barley, rye, almonds, lettuce, apples, figs, asparagus, eggs, cabbage, cucumber, coconuts, walnuts, blueberries, and onions.)

The Virgo Cell Salt:

Potassium sulfate also known as "Kali Suph" is the Virgo tissue cell salt. It helps primarily in the manufacturing and distribution of oily secretions in both the skin and hair. The skin secretions keep the pores open, which ultimately aids in perspiration and the elimination of toxins. Insufficient amounts of potassium sulfate can cause clogging of the pores and buildup of toxins in the epidermal layers of the skin. It is beneficial to use when treating abnormal skin conditions. Potassium sulfate is also an important component of hair and the scalp and can minimize dandruff issues. It carries oxygen to the skin cells and is effective in reducing scar tissue formation and maintaining youthful looking skin. It works extremely well with vitamin E and can be thought of as a lubricant that keeps the body's machinery working efficiently. A lack of potassium sulfate results in a person uncomfortable and eventually suffocated in an overheated environment, especially around noon when the sun is at its peak.

(Potassium sulfate can be found in endive, chicory, carrots, oats, rye, and many salad vegetables.)

The Libra Cell Salt:

Sodium phosphate also known as "Nat Phos" is the Libra tissue cell salt. It maintains the body's acid and alkaline balance by preventing excess acidity or alkalinity, especially in the bloodstream. It aids the kidneys with their normal functions and responsibilities. Too much acidity in the body can cause a person to go into a coma and collapse. In order for the rest of the other cell salts to work properly, the acid and alkaline balance from sodium phosphate must be maintained. Since it removes excess acidity, sodium phosphate has been used to treat gout, kidney stones, tired muscles, ulcers, and acid reflux. Insufficient amounts of sodium phosphate have been shown to produce a yellowish coating on the tongue.

(Sodium phosphate can be found in celery, carrots, spinach, asparagus, apples, figs, strawberries, blueberries, raisins, almonds, fresh coconut, oatmeal, and black or wild rice.)

The Scorpio Cell Salt:

Calcium sulfate also known as "Calc Sulph" is the Scorpio tissue cell salt. It is an important constituent of the cells of all connective tissue and is absolutely essential in all healing processes. All of the sulfate salts have a sanitizing effect on the body. Calcium sulfate is nature's cleanser and purifying agent. This salt prevents the gastric juices from dissolving the lining of the stomach and has bee used to treat ulcers. A shortage of calcium sulfate usually results in stomach problems, and since it is also critical in forming the reproductive hormones, lack of it affects the ovaries, testes and prostate gland. When used in concert with other salts, it is used to alleviate constipation. Whenever old or harmful substances are to be removed from the body, calcium sulfate is recommended to help.

(Calcium sulfate can be found in onions, asparagus, kale, garlic, mustard, cress, turnips, figs, cauliflower, radishes, leeks, prunes, black cherries, gooseberries, blueberries, and coconuts.)

The Sagittarius Cell Salt:

Silicon dioxide also known as Silica is the Sagittarius tissue cell salt. It is one of the most important ingredients in glass and is developed naturally in the body when the lenses of the eyes are formed. It also gives the teeth, bones, fingernails and hair a glossy appearance. Its small but sharp crystals keep the skin pores open. Taking silica after surgery helps minimize scar tissue formation. The body requires only a trace amount of silica to maintain good health, but in its absence we find that the fingernails become brittle and the teeth begin to decay. It is an excellent compliment to the Cancer tissue salt, calcium fluoride.

(Silicon dioxide can be found in the skin of fruits, the outer covering of ancient grains, figs, prunes, and strawberries.)

The Capricorn Cell Salt:

Calcium phosphate also known as "Calc Phos" is the Capricorn tissue cell salt. It is essential to bone tissue and structure. Out of all of the tissue cell salts, the body requires the largest amount from calcium phosphate, especially during childhood growth and development or when recovering from broken bones. It is an essential part of the digestive juices and without a sufficient amount of it, foods can pass through the digestive tract without releasing their nutritional components. Calcium phosphate has an important role in the clothing mechanism of the blood, and an insufficiency can mean that the blood takes longer to coagulate, resulting in hemorrhage. Bright's disease has been found to be related to a lack of this tissue salt, as are skeletal problems like rickets, curvature of the spine, and many tooth complications. Rheumatism, arthritis and swollen or painful joints, like in bursitis, are helped by a daily dose of calcium phosphate. It works well with potassium phosphate and time has shown that they are commonly used together.

(Calcium phosphate can be found in strawberries, plums, blueberries, figs, spinach, asparagus, lettuce, cucumber, almonds, coconut, lentils, brown beans, rye, barley, and sea fish.)

The Aquarius Cell Salt:

Sodium chloride also known as "Nat Mur" is the Aquarius tissue cell salt. It is chemically identifiable to table salt but in a much more natural and highly purified state. Its uses as a preservative and as a seasoning have been known since ancient times. Fruits and vegetables are good natural sources of this salt. It is found in most of the body's cells and fluids, where one of its most important roles is to preserve the proper fluid tensions via osmotic pressure in the cells in order to help them retain their shape. Its primary function is to transport fluids to areas of the body where they are required. Symptoms involving an insufficient amount of sodium chloride are usually associated with water related conditions like colds, dropsy, dryness of the mouth, constipation, shingles and a slowed healing from insect bites. A lack of this salt has been shown to cause insomnia due to the brain tissue being too dry. Too much water in the brain however may cause a heavy, tired and drowsy feeling. Upon awakening you may even feel more tired than when you went to sleep. Sodium chloride is has been helpful in treating blisters, swelling, itching, eczema, redness and sunburns. A paste of sodium chloride, potassium chloride, calcium sulfate, and iron phosphate applied to the skin has been shown to be effective in the relief of skin problems and itching from insect bites. With the exception of calcium phosphate, we need more sodium chloride than the other tissue cell salts.

(Sodium chloride can be found in strawberries, apples, figs, spinach, cabbage, lettuce, chestnuts, coconuts, and lentils.)

The Pisces Cell Salt:

Iron phosphate also known as "Ferrum Phos" is the Pisces tissue cell salt. This is the only common metal salt among the twelve cell salts and it is extremely important due to its ability to make all of the other cell salts more effective. It is required for healthy red blood cells and a lack of it can cause anemia. Its most important function is to distribute oxygen to all of the body's tissues, which is especially imperative when the body is fighting off infection. Insufficient oxygen levels means that all basic body processes slow down. The lack of ferrum phosphate can cause an individual to become tired quickly. This cell salt is essential in treating many afflictions because it supplies the increased oxygen needed by suffering tissues. It shortens the period of recovery and promotes more rapid healing. All living cells require oxygen to produce energy for all of their chemical reactions, making this tissue cell salt absolutely essential.

(Iron phosphate can be found in lettuce, strawberries, radishes, horseradish, spinach, lentils, and cabbage.)

Ch.24: More On Our Universe

The force and power of the universe is both in us and around is. It is up to us to become and remain aware of it and to harness it in the most productive ways possible. The more we are responsible for our energy the easier it is to manage it and to reap the benefits from it.

The Sirius star system is located in the constellation of *Canis Minor*, the "Little Dog" in the southern portion of the heavens near the constellations Orion and Canis Major, the "Big Dog". Sirius resides in the celestial sea at 15 degrees below the celestial equator, at about 23 degrees in the sign of Cancer. Sirius B is the central sun that the Sun in our solar system orbits around. As a result of this, Sirius B governs the rotation and orbital cycles of our Sun, our neighboring planets, as well as planet Earth. It is an excellent celestial system to study in order to gain a better understanding of how we function down here as humans.

The Sirius star system is profound and its function is replicated all throughout the universe. Sirius B is the oldest of the stars and its name means "deep beginning". The ancients described it as the reservoir and source of all things in this realm. It is the smallest and yet the heaviest star in creation. Its spin orientation is the cosmic foundation for the organization and motion of the other stars and planets in the universe. Its movement keeps all other stars in their respective places and without its extremely intense magnetic field none of them would be able to remain in place. Sirius B forces them to keep their trajectory. Their existence is also made possible by the hydrogen it ejects out into the rest of space. It's outer atmosphere is said to have been released into space millions of years ago. Sirius B is labeled as a dwarf star that has completed the cycle of regular star life.

Sirius A is a younger star and appears to be blue in color, as more youthful stars tend to vibrate in the blue light spectrum. This is due to the fact that younger stars burn hotter and in most cases appear to shine brighter than others. Sirius A has much of its hydrogen pulled back into the strong gravitational pull of Sirius B. The hydrogen essence of Sirius A however is thrown off of Sirius B due to its extremely fast rotation. This hydrogen essence from Sirius A is then hurled into space and much of it is showered down into our solar system in the form of ultra violet light. The Dogon tribe, from Mali in North Africa, teaches that this stream of ionized hydrogen from the Sirius system is purifying to the Sun and planet Earth.

Sirius C is invisible to the naked eye and can go undetected without the appropriate technology or level of consciousness needed to identify it. Sirius C is considered to be feminine in nature and is described in different African cultures as the "Great Mystery". Some modern astrologers believe that this star has made its way into our solar system and that this is a sign fulfilling ancient prophecies. The relationship between Sirius A and Sirius B is the heavenly version of the man and woman here on earth. The woman can produce a male or female which is the terrestrial version of Sirius B sustaining herself as well as feeding hydrogen ions to Sirius A, who responds by impregnating her with the hydrogen ions siphoned back into the orbit of Sirius B and then out into the universe giving birth to other forms of creation in the same way a man would impregnate a woman soon followed by her delivering a new life on Earth.

In outer space, both stars and H2 regions are examples of hydrogen plasma. In physics, plasma is described as a gaseous body that has an organized and congruent molecular makeup. This plasma can be explained as crystalized gas. The molecules in the plasma maintain an abundance of circulating free electrons and since plasma has an abundance of these electrons, physicists even refer to plasma as "ionized gas." In space, hydrogen plasma has been shown to be the main fuel source of all main sequence stars and is also what causes H2 clouds to emit an ultraviolet halo. All stars are born in H2 regions.

The regular gas form of hydrogen is called a H1 region. These are nebula masses of hydrogen that are not yet ionized or charged. Because of this, H1 regions do not emit ultraviolet light like plasma. Stars are not born in H1 regions either. These areas are composed of hydrogen in its colder state and it remains inert. This is an excellent example of the power of warmth and how temperature plays a role in mediating matter.

In astrophysics, concentrated blackness manifest as ionized hydrogen plasma (H2). This is the primary fuel source for our galaxy as well as what we know of the other portions of the universe. For Earth, there are several major sources of ionized hydrogen. A main one is the black hole at the galactic core, which is located at 26 degrees Sagittarius from Earth's point of view. The spirals that spin out of this galactic core define the shape of our galaxy and are what we see when looking at visuals of the Milky Way. The hydrogen ions rain down on our planet from here in the form of ultraviolet light (blackness). Another source is the H2 nebulae, which can be described as space clouds of ionized hydrogen. These hydrogen clouds are the birthplace of stars.

There are many who try to discredit the science of astrology but this is simply due to varying degrees of ignorance. The home of the vice president of the United States of America is at the United States Naval Observatory. This is where the stars and planets are observed with the most advanced and finest forms of technology in order to map out the current and future energetic patterns caused by celestial movements. This is one of the oldest agencies in the United States and its function is to produce positioning, navigation, and timing (PNT) so that those running the country can improve upon their decision-making. After these stellar observations are made, the government via the vice president is instructed on how to carry on according to what is in their best interest. If astronomy and astrology were not significant, then the so-called 2nd most powerful man on the western hemisphere would not be living there.

The Eternal Present Moment

"I have only just a minute..

Only sixty seconds in it..

Forced up on me..

Cant refuse it..

Didn't seek it..

Didn't choose it..

But its up to me to use it..

I must suffer if I lose it..

Give a count if I abuse it..

Just a tiny little minute..

But eternity is in it.."

By: Benjamin E. Mays

No matter the time of day or the circumstance we find ourselves in, every single moment that we experience occurs in the now. Being present plays a huge role in becoming healthy because it allows for us to genuinely address life at any given moment. We always have an opportunity to come correct and do things better than before because all the seemingly new moments are created in the now. When we are not fully present to what is going on within us or outside of us, we set ourselves up for failure. We experience anxiety when we are too concerned with future events and we experience depression when we allow past circumstances and events to weigh us down. Staying present automatically empowers us by giving us the opportunity to choose how we will handle any situation. Being in the moment also allows for us to stay on schedule when it comes to the natural order and pace of the universe. We know these patterns and cycles unconsciously but here is a quick review:

The Eternal Present Moment

Seconds

Minutes

Hours

Days

Weeks

Months

Seasons

Years

Decades

Centuries

Millennia

Dispensations

This is a blueprint that we can trust and use to plan our affairs with. If you haven't noticed by now, the universe is divinely organized and it is up to us to stay in line and in tune with this reality and if we fail to do so then we consciously or unconsciously call for our own undesirable consequences.

"To every thing there is a season, and a time to every purpose under the heaven."

-Ecclesiastes 3:1

Ch.25: Calendars and Timing

Egyptian/Kemetic	Modern
Sekhert	Seconds
Min	Minutes
Heru/Horus	Hours
Re (Ra)	Days
Mut	Months
Anu	Annual
Nun	Noon
Nut	Night

The original Egyptian/Kemetic calendar was a multifaceted system used to track astronomical and astrological phenomena. It was designed to keep track of different cycles in nature so that the priests and kings could better coordinate the affairs of their homelands with the cycles of nature. Many Egyptologist claim that Egyptian culture began with the 1st dynasty of Menes between 3100 BCE-4240 BCE however there are Egyptian/Kemetic accounts of their history dating back tens of thousands of years before the Fist Dynasty was founded. Seek out the *Royal Papyrus of Turin* to learn more about this neglected history. It has listed many of the Kings who ruled Egypt/Kemet from Menes through the New Kingdom of the 18th Dynasty and also the rule of at least ten different Neter who reigned on the planet prior to the first mention of Menes.

Prior to what we refer to as 1582 there was no such thing as the past as we know it. There was no A.D. or B.C. until the adoption of the Gregorian calendar, which was invented by Aloysius Lilius and Christopher Clavius both of whom were commissioned by Pope Gregory the 13th. Prior to that Julius Caesar had commissioned an Egyptian astronomer and priest by the name of Sosigenes to develop the Julian calendar, which was modeled after the Egyptian/Kemetic count of days. This occurred in so called 45 B.C. The Julian calendar was slightly modified in 382 CE by Emperor Constantine. He is credited historically with the world's adoption of the seven-day week and the four-week month in order to better incorporate Christian symbolism into the Roman calendar system. The year 0 CE of the Julian and Gregorian calendars corresponds with the shifting of the equinox sunrise from the sign of Aries to the sign of Pisces. This was also falsely associated with the birth of Jesus as promoted by the Abrahamic mythos.

Before these two recent calendar updates, we for the most part lived in the eternal present moment and respected the universe as one all-inclusive stage for eternity to express itself thru. With this knowledge of history it becomes easier to understand that as long as we continue to live fragmented and separate ourselves from the past and future, we will inevitably create some form of suffering. A solution to this would be to live in the eternal present moment recognizing that we are all individually and collectively causers of reality by how we choose to be responsible with what exists right now.

For the past few hundred years, we witnessed the western world flood the world with false historical narratives that made it seem as though the people who currently occupy the world's hoods or black and brown communities are powerless and have no significance. The truth is that the past and the future does not exist in the manner that we were taught. What we refer to as the future is the change taking place in and around you in the ever present now. When we begin to rule our minds in the present moment we can begin to better rule our personal worlds. Time is essentially how we measure changes in our magnetic fields.

Ch.26: The Sun Comes First

We rely on the Sun for everything and the quality of our relationship with it plays an undeniable and essential role when it comes to our health. We need it to tell time and also to grow the foods we eat. We trust it to wake us up in the mornings and to sustain us with its vital energies. It serves as one of the best teachers known to man as it continuously gives without asking us for anything. Everything comes second to the Sun as it is the primary representative of the creator on this plane.

We have accepted the idea of time outside of us but many of us are unfamiliar with how it more realistically occurs inside of us. The magnetism of the Earth along with the stimulating forces of the Sun cause constant but orderly changes in us. These internal fluctuations have become known as chronobiology and scientists are still making discoveries regarding this field to this day. Chronobiology is a field of science that examines timing processes in living organisms via biological rhythms. There are four main types but in this text we will highlight the circadian rhythm, as it is the most relevant to our discussion here on health. The Sun however is responsible for all them as it is both the manufacturer and stimulator of the human body.

Biological Rhythms	
Diurnal Rhythms	Similar to the circadian rhythm but synched with day and night
Ultradian Rhythms	lasting shorter than a 24 hour period and at a higher frequency
Infradian Rhythms	lasting longer than a 24 hours period like a menstrual cycle
Circadian Rhythms	A 24 hour cycle that includes physiological and behavioral patterns

The ethmoid organ, which is tuned into the lines of geomagnetic force, has the largest amount of natural loadstones crystals in our body. It picks up geomagnetic micropulsations coming off the surface of the earth that naturally set the circadian and ultradian cycles of the body.

The circadian clock inside of us responds to light and darkness and has a physical, mental, and behavioral influence on us. It helps to regulate functions in us so that we remain in balance and in sync with the universe around us. The most popular functions are the secretion of melatonin and serotonin. Melatonin production is stimulated in response to darkness and is naturally secreted by the pineal gland. It is the main hormone involved with sleep. Serotonin is a precursor to melatonin and is produced from tryptophan. Serotonin is referred to as the daytime hormone and is secreted in response to light whether it be natural or artificial. Tryptophan is an essential amino acid that creates nitrogen balance in the body and also plays a vital role in the production of niacin, which is essential in creating the neurotransmitter serotonin.

Functions and Patterns Regulated by Our Internal Clock
Sleep schedule
Appetite
Body temperature
Hormone levels
Alertness
Daily performance
Blood pressure
Reaction times

In order to honor these patterns it is best to mimic the actions of the sun in our daily affairs i.e. rise when the sun comes up in the morning, give our best efforts during the day, and rest when the sun goes down at the end of the day. If we do otherwise we can expect to suffer from a variety of issues related to our internal rhythms. Some of the most popular problems to come about as a result from not mirroring the sun are anxiety, getting tired during the day, depression, low performance in the workplace, being more prone to accidents, a decrease in alertness, and an increased risk for diabetes and obesity.

Acupuncture, reflexology, and acupressure can used to rebalance a person if they have not been honoring these cycles and find themselves suffering from any of the mentioned issues but eventually a change in schedule will be needed in order to sustain the balance. If we are not addressing the cause of the problems we suffer from then we cannot expect to heal from them. Temporary solutions and quick fixes will only add on to the problems at hand so always be sure to seek out the root of the troubles you may find yourself dealing with.

Recommended Habits to Help us Harmonize with the Sun	
5-7 am	Wake up to gratitude and using the restroom if possible
7-9 am	Drink water, have early morning sex or go for a walk
9-11 am	Review plans for the day and visualize them while your energy is at its peak
11-1 pm	Eat some fruit or drink a smoothie to nourish your cells
1-3 pm	Study or work and allow for your food to assimilate
3-5 pm	Continue to work or study
5-7 pm	Eat a healthy snack or a final meal
7-9 pm	Do some light reading and get a foot massage or reflexology session
9-11 pm	Calm socializing and sex with your spouse or loved one
11-1 am	Soothing music to help with sleep and restoration
1-3 am	Deep sleep to detox the liver and blood
3-5 am	Deep sleep to detox the lungs

Organ & Peak Performance Times

Organ	Peak Performance	Rest State
Lungs	3 AM	3 PM
Large Intestines	5 AM	5 PM
Stomach	7 AM	7 PM
Spleen	9 AM	9 PM
Heart	11 AM	11 PM
Small Intestine	1 PM	1 AM
Bladder	3 PM	3 AM
Kidneys	5 PM	5 AM
Heart Protector	7 PM	7 AM
Triple Burner	9 PM	9 AM
Gall Bladder	11 PM	11 AM
Liver	1 AM	1 PM

The organs of the human body are subject to the cycles, seasons, and rhythms of the universe. There is a universal harmony that compliments and blends all things. The universal energy travels through every part of the body and concentrates itself in the organs, glands and bodily systems. Each organ has a two hour window where this universal energy surges through it the most and also a corresponding two hour window when the organs are in a state of rest. Exercises can be performed and nutrition can be consumed at any time of the day, however eating or exercising during the peak hours of an organ's energy flow will prove to be the most effective period for best results.

We use the Sun to tell time and it determines our internal activities. There is no way we can get around dealing with it on any day. Light is all there is down here on this level of existence. The Sun is the manufacturer of the physical body and must be respected in order to achieve and maintain true states of health It is the supreme provider of life and is the greatest source of energy present within our solar system. Water is known to many cultures as the source of life and yet the Sun is the source of all water. We trigger different biological processes when we expose various parts of the body to sunlight. For example, when the reproductive area is exposed the Sun, hormone levels can be multiplied by up to 300% depending on the quality of the body and the condition of the region the person is in. Likewise, exposing areas of the face and head to sunlight stimulates our brain's pineal and hypothalamus glands to produce neurotransmitters that support overall mental functioning. One of the greatest health myths is that the sun is detrimental to one's health and is responsible for causing the body to produce cancer cells.

Sunlight Electrifies The Air

As sunlight passes through our atmosphere, it electrically charges some of the air molecules, typically in a ratio of 4:5 negative to positive ions. Some of the negative ions are oxygen ions while carbon dioxide ions contribute to the positive ions along with other gases. These numbers fluctuate of course depending on the environment so a city or urban area like Detroit may have less hydrogen ions than a place like the amazon rainforest where oxygen is heavily produced from the abundance of plants and trees. Other factors in our natural environment like radioactivity in the soil or air, thunderstorms, and the active movement of water through the air like areas with waterfalls contribute to the production of ions as well.

If the number of positive ions increase with a corresponding decrease in negative ions, a person may feel adverse effects like a headache, nasal obstruction, hoarseness, fatigue, dry throat, or even dizziness. An increase in negative ions on the other hand produces feelings of exhilaration and well-being. Positively charged air depresses the adrenal glands and their ability to secret hormone that protect the body against stress. This means that living or working too often indoors can leave people vulnerable to stress unless the outside negatively charged air is allowed to come in through an open window, a door, or is properly balanced by an up to par heating or air conditioning unit. Negatively charged air increases the mucus flow and speeds up the rate at which cilia move, while positively charge air does the polar opposite. It is important that we keep the film of mucus moving so that germs and bacteria can be expelled properly as opposed to multiplying and invading the body resulting in bronchitis or pneumonia.

On Sunlight and Skin

Sunlight triggers the synthesis of vitamins inside the body after interacting with our melanin. When UVB rays hit human skin, they cooperate with what is called the 7-DHC proteins there in order to produce vitamin D3. 7-DHC is a precursor to cholesterol that is photochemically converted in our skin. This process varies in intensity according to the amount and quality of melanin that one possesses. While people with certain genetic dispositions may get sunburns and even skin cancer from too much sun exposure, the more original people with darker hues tend to absorb and trap the sunlight, which is converted into nutrients for the rest of the body to benefit from. Suntans are popular for darkening the complexion of ones skin but what is actually taking place is the body increasing its hue in order to attract and house more light. The darker a person is, the more they are able to interact with the Sun and its forces. This ability however can be altered when one consumes too many unnatural substances i.e. white sugars, manufactured foods, genetically modified foods, etc.

More Health Benefits of Sunlight
Sunlight encourages healthy circulation and blood flow
Sunlight stimulates the production of red blood cells
Sunlight exposure can lower blood pressure
Sunlight increases the body's energy levels
Sunlight prevents vitamin D deficiencies
Sunlight reduces the risk of cancer
Sunlight improves moods and mental states
Sunlight improves sleeping patterns
Sunlight helps with weight loss
Sunlight increases eye health
Sunlight improves bone integrity and structure

Chlorophyll from Sunlight

Chlorophyll is responsible for giving plants the green hue we are familiar with. It is a pigment and a compound that helps plants to absorb and transform sunlight as they undergo the process of photosynthesis. Chlorophyll is found in most plants and in the leaves of fruits to greater or lesser degrees. The greener the plant is the greater the concentration of chlorophyll. It has a tremendous amount of health benefits for the human body and can even be used in combination with quality sources of iron to replenish and build of healthy red blood cells. Some of the greatest sources of chlorophyll are green leafy vegetables, blue-green algae, phytoplankton and sprouts.

The Different Types of Chlorophyll	
Chlorophyll A	Absorbs light in the blue-violet region and reflects green
Chlorophyll B	Absorbs red-blue light and reflects green
Chlorophyll C	Found in brown algae and diatoms
Chlorophyll D	Found in red algae
Bacteriochlorophyll	Absorbs red or far red light and is found in heliobacteria

Sodium copper chlorophyllin is a derivative of chlorophyll and is both water-soluble and bioavailable. The antioxidant capacity of chlorophyllin is about 2000 times greater than blueberries and 20 times greater than resveratrol, which is an organic molecule known as one the best tools for fighting against oxidative damages caused by carcinogens and radiation.

Health Benefits of Chlorophyll
Chlorophyll detoxes and nourishes the blood simultaneously
Chlorophyll helps to promote the production of red blood cells
Chlorophyll is an all natural body deodorizer
Chlorophyll has anti cancer properties
Chlorophyll has anti inflammatory properties
Chlorophyll can assist in the healing of wounds if applied topically
Chlorophyll improves the liver's ability to remove waste from the body
Chlorophyll increase the energy of the body as it is a form of secondhand sunlight
Chlorophyll assist with hormonal balance

The hemoglobin in our blood and chlorophyll have very similar molecular structures. The difference is that hemoglobin is built around iron (Fe) while chlorophyll is built around magnesium (Mg). Chlorophyll even helps to do the job of hemoglobin when it is ingested. He primary function of hemoglobin is to transport oxygen from the lungs to the rest of the body. This is one of the many ways that the law of correspondence shows up revealing our affinity with the universe around us.

The Sun and You

We have discussed light but want to reemphasize that it is eternal. What we know of, as life is simply the alteration of its forms. We are taught by western education that it has a speed but the truth is that light has a rate of induction. It is already everywhere and is only activated by magnetic forces, pressure mediation and conductors. Photons were supposedly the smallest components of life but breakthroughs and rediscoveries in physics has proven that they are the portion of the light that we able to perceive at any given moment when the proper technologies are used. What we refer to as photons can change their color (or frequency) depending on how many of them are present. For now we can describe them as the purest form of energy. When one seemingly unites with a second photon through resonance, they temporarily become a particle. Electrons are said to capture energetic photons emitted from the fission of the Sun through resonance. They are also said to be in a continuous motion and to have their own wavelength with a particular oscillation and resonance just like a radio receiver. As particles they have their own length and that gives them their own frequency. They are essentially the final fundamental expression of matter, materialized as water in our bodies.

Sunlight is an underestimated form of nutrition. Sunlight alone is known to activate over two hundred enzymes into action. Electron rich foods from our sun give the cells what they require the most and result in us not needing as much food as the average person. The pineal gland is commonly called the first or third eye and acts like a lens that responds to light s brightness and color. The pineal gland is responsible for all inner light activities. Light is transformed at the skin but enters the body mostly through the eyes and heads directly to the pineal gland to be mediated for our body's use. This light is made to be bioavailable in the form of colloids or crystalizes eventually into minerals if it is not reserved as raw energy

Colloids are captured and stored during the photosynthesis process. As discussed earlier, they have their origin in the stars and cosmic dust and provide fuel for all living beings on our planet. There is an inexhaustible and free source of energy stored in the cosmic rays and in the ethers around us. Plants and fruits tap into this energy that has been drawn from the fission reaction of the celestial objects, stars, and our local sun. The cosmic energy through constant densification forms the material we see in our universe.

There are many forms of energy found in our universe. There is a specific type of energy however found in extraordinary healing known as radiant energy. It is in both the sun and our physical bodies as one can be thought of as the inverse of the other. We may appear to be solidified beings to the naked eye but science has proven that we radiate energy from the inside on out that can extend feet away from the parameters created by our skin. In the presence of the Sun's rays, electrons in our skin become stored within the interplay of the fatty acid and protein complex. Taking solar electrons into this lipoprotein heightens and maintains our sense of well-being.

Section 5 Summary

What Asa detailed in section 5 is how God painted the perfect masterpiece, referring to the universe, specifically outer space. Every celestial body, and its movement affect what, who, and why we are as humans. Every stroke of God's brush beams our physical features, personalities, diet recommendations, and more. Our terrestrial landscape is a product of celestial matter so we are definitely connected to the skies like we are the earth.

Understanding this connection, we must know that while much of what we research about optimal physical health can be accurate – physical exercise, proper nutrition, sleep, hygiene, etc., those tangibles must be met with sometimes subtle intangibles – the sun, chemical reactions in the ether and our bodies, our locations and environments, mental exercising and conditioning, and other phenomenon we don't ever consider when we think about what's needed to be completely healthy. Reality is, the art piece that God has painted dictates that optimal health comes from a healthy spirit – being connected to the source (religion describes the source as God), a healthy mind which crafts our reality as we see fit, and a healthy body which is required to house all this divine power that's within all of us. In all, health starts with the spirit first, the mind next, resulting in the body following.

In this world of commercial health, fitness, and nutrition, we must know the difference between activities that make us look good, activities that make us feel good, and activities that ensure we are walking in our divinity daily which will certainly have us looking and feeling good too. Optimal health rains down from the heavens and is planted into the earth for us to soak up both the sky and the ground.

Black Is Gold, and the Color Spectrum

Ch.27 Color Is Vibration

On Pigments

Chlorophyll is just one of the pigments that nourish us and allows for us to experience the wonders latent in creation. While vitamins, minerals, and other popular sources of nutrients are household names, the pigments play a very crucial role in our wellbeing and serve us as essential sources of nourishment that we can't seem to find elsewhere. In biology pigments are also referred to as biochromes and are described as substances that have color resulting from selective light absorption. Some of these are naturally occurring in the body while others can be found in plants and fruits.

Pigments and their Roles

Pigments	Role
Hemoglobin	Oxygen transfer from lungs to tissues
Neuroglobin	Increases oxygen availability to brain
Cytoglobin	Transfer of oxygen from arteries to brain
Myoglobin	Facilitates oxygen diffusion
Pheomelanin	Imparts yellowish and reddish colors
Black Eumealin	Darker Skin Pigmentation
Brown Eumelanin	Lighter Skin Pigmentation
Bluish Neuromelanin	Substantia Nigra
Black Neuromelanin	Locus Coeruleus
Neuropsin	Governs synaptic plasticity
Photopsin	Signal feedback to photoreceptors
Melanopsin	Helps to set circadian rhythms
Rhodopsin	Visual phototransduction
Lutein	Light filter for protecting eye tissues
Zeaxanthin	Eye integrity
Panopsin (Opsin 3)	Negative regulator of melanogenesis
Chromosomes	Exclusive genetics and transportation

Ch.28: On Melanin

Melanin is a color pigment composed of a hydrocarbon chain which has various amino (nitrogen based) compounds attached to it. Carbon is responsible for the blackness we are familiar with when observing melanin. Carbon is the organizing molecule that gives melanin its structure. Carbon also gives melanin the ability to absorb energy and bind with other molecules while retaining stability and coherence. Besides carbon, the two elements that are essential to the structure of melanin are copper and sulfur. Copper is incorporated into the melanin molecule via the amino acid tyrosine.

Tyrosinase is an organic and metallic amino compound that is organized around carbon, nitrogen, and copper. It is a catalyst for melanin reproduction and is the amino compound that facilitates melanin's capacity to conduct different types of frequencies. Sulfur on the other hand is incorporated into the melanin molecule through an amino acid called cysteine. Cysteine is an amino compound that is organized around carbon, nitrogen, and sulfur. It allows for melanin to create or release heat, as it is needed for the body. Cysteine also cleanses and purifies melanin by removing toxic elements that have been absorbed into melanin. This chemical masterpiece is still being studied till this day as more discoveries are constantly being made.

21 Facts about Melanin
Melanin is a pigment found in the skin & various internal organs
Melanin is composed of hydrocarbon chains & various amino compounds
Melanin is a complex biopolymer
Melanin is found in the nuclei of cells
Melanin is the central compound in the body
Melanin governs neurological and hormonal activities in the body
Melanin can turn light into ionic food for the body
Melanin absorbs & utilizes cosmic, ultra-violet, & infrared waves
Melanin functions like a localized computer
Melanin analyzes external conditions and initiates bodily responses
Melanin discharges electrical impulses from heat and pressure from sound waves
Melanin is a conductor of the body's ionic charge and acts like a battery for the body
Melanin conducts the electrochemical exchanges from the body's electrolytes
Melanin can alter its frequency to match and vibrate in unison with an external one
Melanin is condensed dark matter
Melanin is essential for all sentient beings
Melanin is self regenerating
Melanin is the most biological equivalent to love
Melanin exist on all planets and meteors
Melanin is the most divine substance found in the human body
Melanin is the most capable and adaptable substance known to man

More On Melanin

In his book *Dark Light Consciousness,* Dr. Edward Bruce Bynum, who is the clinical psychologist and director of behavioral medicine at University of Massachusetts at Amherst, tracked the evolution of the human brain whereby he explains that dark matter on the exterior of the brain improved its ability to capture light. *"We see that over time there is a gradual increase in its capacity to absorb light. This is because there is an increasing darkness that covers its surface. This darkness gives it the capacity to absorb light."* He describes the brain as having a threefold structure, which includes the reptilian brain stem, the midbrain of the limbic system, and the highly developed neocortex. The evolutionary marvel in the brain is pretty complex and seems to have something to do with the presence of neuromelanin (melanin in the brain) and its ability to "fold space" as Bynum describes it. Melanin, not to be confused with melatonin, is made by cells called melanocytes, which provide pigmentation to skin, eyes, and hair. Melatonin, on the other hand, is involved in the synchronization of the circadian rhythm of physiological functions and sleep. It is secreted from the pineal gland when one is submerged in darkness. Neuromelanin is highly sensitive to subtle forms of EM activity and is believed to be the primary factor contributing to the advancements of the brain. Bynum also states the following: *"Beyond the brain and brain stem, this melanin is represented in ample amounts in our internal organs...heart, lungs, kidneys, and gastro-intestinal tract, all contained in a structure bounded by skin. Melanin is able to...shift energy, from one state to another, from vibration to sound, to heat, to light. Since all forms of energy are related to each other it is not difficult to see that the subtle energy field of the body referred to in the esoteric traditions as...the energy body, the etheric body, the light or luminous body...is connected to an energy field that may partially be generated by the bioelectrical capacities of melanin in and on the surface of our inner organs is partially why we believe that the sensitive human nervous system can detect geodynamic forces arising from within the Erath."* While everyone possesses different states and degrees of melanin, this conversation is relevant as it reveals the significance of what we were born with and why we should go about protecting it ad nourishing it via our diet and lifestyle.

Melanin has a tetrahedral shape, which is the same as the pyramids, and this is noteworthy as this geometry is essential for conduction at some of the highest levels possible. Melanocytes are mature melanin forming cells found concentrated in large amounts in the bottom layer of the skin's epidermis, the uvea (middle layer of the eye), the inner ear, vaginal epithelium, meninges, bones, and especially in the heart. Melanosomes are organelles found in our cells that serve as a site for synthesis, storage and transportation of melanin. Melanogenesis is the complex process our body uses to produce melanin in the melanosomes by melanocytes. We are most familiar with the visible color spectrum but blackness goes thru its own phases inside of us as well as in the universe around us. Melanin is the medium that the cosmic blackness uses to go thru its processes.

Blackness

We have been bombarded with western education's depiction of black being evil, undesirable, ugly, etc. however this was done by design and could not be further from the truth. Blackness is the most powerful force in creation. The tone of black in the visible light spectrum is the sum total of all colors combined. Black is known to absorb all lights of the color spectrum and is also the source that they are derived from. A great analogy would be the zero in the number system as it is not truly empty but is the source of all the numbers. Blackness is also the true hue of ultraviolet. It is the tone of the cosmic substance responsible for matter.

Western science makes it seem as though only bad scenarios are possible from increased ultraviolet light/blackness on our planet. Mainly people of European decent are concerned with this but this is because their bodies are not equipped to handle the vibrations entering our atmosphere at this time. Their bodies burn, mutate, and breakdown when expose to frequencies outside of toleration range. Destruction is a feature of some phases of the process of blackening but this is only for things that are no longer useful to the overall benefit of the universe. Blackness is actually something that we should begin to revere and to appreciate, as it is responsible for our successes and experiences.

Substantia Nigra

The human brain is encased inside of blackness and yet the Substantia Nigra is the still the darkest portion inside of this closed space. It means black substance in Latin. This is apart of the midbrain that produces dopamine involved in bodily movement and performance. The Substantia Nigra is made of two distinct regions i.e. the pars compacta where it gets its dark coloring from the large number of dopamine neurons as they express high levels of a dark pigment called neuromelanin and pars reticulata which is more heavily populated with GABA neurons. Magnetism is also one of the key features of this part of the brain. Many cognitive diseases are manifested when the Substantia Nigra is impaired. It is a biological testament to the power and potential of blackness as its functions are essential for the rest of the body to function properly. Its hue allows for it to communicate with the deep regions and portions of our universe, as they are made available for our bodies to follow suit after.

Black Body Radiation

Max Planck, 1858-1947, is known as the originator of quantum theory. He isn't given due credit for his contributions in the western educational system because of the nature of the discoveries he made and the time period in which he made them in. While quantum physics and theory are popular now amongst other things, Planck's most significant but underestimated contribution was the coining of the term *black body radiation*. A black body according to physics is an idealized physical body that absorbs all forms of electromagnetic radiation regardless of frequency or the angle of incidence. The name black body is used because it "absorbs" radiation from all frequencies and is able to "emit" them as well. As his findings became plausible and were eventually shown to be factual, they were also swept under the radar and away from the public eye because if publicized, the world would see how naturally powerful and capable the original people of the planet are and that alone would be yet another obvious reason to put a dent in global systematic white supremacy. Even though it was considered an idealized body, it sparked too much attention at the time and raised brows as its more physically relevant properties began to be the crux of conversations.

Ch.29: On Colors and Nutrition

While pigments may be known by their colors, there is a science to hues and theirs respective contributions. Notice how the colors inside the visible spectrum seem to get lighter as we go from red to green and darker as we go from green to purple. In Mother Nature both darkness and light are equally important. Colors can be altered when vibratory rates are changed or they can be combined mathematically to produce different shades. Red (action) when balanced with blue (clear mental picture) results in purple (partaking in celestial instruction). We can observe the color spectrum as a linear band or we can view it as a circle making its way through the process of blackening. Notice how red and blue appear to be on opposing ends of the spectrum and how purple serves as a bridge between them.

Black is all encompassing and represents the aspect of nature where all things have their origin. Dark colored foods provide us with both a wide variety of nutrients as well as rare potent forms of nutrition that are too strong to appear as any other hue. *Red* and *orange* colored vegetables supply the body with carotenoids and xanthophylls. *Yellow* colored vegetables provide the body with catechines, isoflavones, lutein, and zeaxanthin. *Green* foods indicate the presence of chlorophyll, which is considered to be the king of antioxidants. Chlorophyll rich foods like chlorella, alfalfa, and cilantro cleanse the blood and promote circulation in the body. If flesh is present in ones diet, it would be wise to pair it with some form of greenery as chlorophyll binds to carcinogens. *Blue* and *purple* colored vegetables supply our bodies with anthocyanins, hydroxystilbenes, and phenols. *Brown* and *white* (not to be confused with manufactured or processed) colored vegetables provide the body with allicin, lignins, and tannins. Remember that everything in existence has a particular rate of vibration and we see here that those of the minerals found in different vegetables determine the color we see when they are grown.

Cells are light sensitive so colored light affects their growth and the manner in which they behave which causes subtle and gentle biochemical changes to take place. Every color we see has a special power, quality, and essence. They can all be used in healing to amplify or balance energy in a person in general or in specific locations in the body. The colors don't just nourish our cells and organs. They have a powerful influence on our emotion states and can come from the foods we eat and even the clothes we wear. When choosing your internal or external color selections, be sure to keep in mind that each choice comes with its own unique vibration and outcome.

Colorimetry is the name of the main science used to measure colors. Another method of color measurement that is significant enough to mention here is spectrophotometry, which is used to identify the light and its wavelengths present in the subject being analyzed or studied. Chromaticity refers to the quality of color associated with hue and saturation as opposed to brightness and lightness. Understanding the colors and their corresponding vibratory rates will prove to be beneficial when one is striving to heal themselves or someone is working will patients who desire help on their personal journey back to wholeness.

Color	Wavelength (nm)	Frequency (Hz)	Energy (eV)
Red	625-740 nm	405-480 THz	1.65-2.00 eV
Orange	590-625 nm	480-510 THz	2.00-2.10 eV
Yellow	565-590 nm	510-530 THz	2.10-2.17 eV
Green	500-565 nm	530-600 THz	2.25-2.34 eV
Blue	540-500 nm	600-680 THz	2.48-2.75 eV
Purple	380-460 nm	680-790 THz	2.95-3.10 eV

Wavelengths are measured in nanometers. They are defined as the spatial period of a wave or the distance between consecutive corresponding points of the same phase of a wave like two adjacent crests or troughs. The inverse of a wavelength is referred to as a spatial frequency. The shorter the wavelength is the greater the power associated with the subject being measured.

Frequency is measured in hertz (Hz), which is equal to one event per second. An easy way to understand frequency is to think of how many times a circle or an objective can be done in a given amount of time. You frequent the restroom more when you drink a lot of water or you frequent the grocery store less when your refrigerator is full. The higher the frequency is the more power is made available.

Energy is what everything is made up of essential and can be described as the potential for work being done or manifestation. It is measured in joules or electron volts (eV) which is the work potentially done by an electron or an apparent singular current of expressed dielectricity.

Far infrared radiation is the band of EM radiation that is longer in wavelength than the red of the visible spectrum. It is responsible for the transmission of radiant heat and is used in physiotherapy to warm tissues, improve circulation, and reduce pain.

Color is simply what the creator chose to differentiate between visible vibrations. The law of vibrations teaches us that nothing rests and that everything moves.

Ch.30: Everything Vibrates

Here we want to take a look specifically at how the law of vibration expresses itself in the human body. When we see the abbreviation MHz it means on million cycles per second. The abbreviation MHz stands for mega hertz.

In the early 1900s, there was a gentleman by the name of Bruce Tainio, who was a student and a researcher in the field of quantum physics. He invented a device called the BT2 Frequency Monitoring System, which was designed to measure the bioelectric frequency of essential oils. He eventually upgraded the system and used it to measure the frequencies of the human body. Notice how a body that is considered to be healthy manages to stay within a certain vibratory range while dis-ease shows up when we allow our vibrations to drop. His research and data showed the following:

In a Healthy Body

The known genius brain vibrates between 80-82 MHz

The brain frequency range is between 72-90 MHz

The average brain vibrates at about 72 MHz

The average human body vibrates between 62-78 MHz

The average thyroid and parathyroid gland vibrate between 62-68 MHz

The average thymus gland vibrates between 65-68 MHz

The average heart vibrates between 67-70 MHz

The average set of lungs vibrates between 58-65 MHz

The average liver vibrates between 55-60 MHz

The average pancreas vibrates between 60-80 MHz

In a Dis-eased Body

Colds and the flu start about 57-60 MHz

Most diseases start around 58 MHz

Candida growth starts at 55 MHz

Cancer cells start at about 42 MHz

Foods and environments have vibratory rates and can be measured as well with more up to date technologies. It is important to keep this in mind when striving to bring restoration and balance back to the body. Remember that the universe is mental and wherever there in mind, energy is present there. Everything that we know of exists in a field of energy. All atoms are an expression of a force that is antecedent to physicality. This means that while we have external means of addressing our different matters that need healing, our priority should be in seeking the powers that exist inside of us.

Nikola Tesla stated that if we could eliminate certain outside frequencies that interfered with out bodies, we could have greater resistance towards disease.

Zero point is where two equal and opposing waves of vibration cancel each other out. Zero point causes vacuum. What is left over is referred to as residuum vibration. This vibration is a reflection of vitality and potential. This extremely fine vibration is a resonance that is nonpolar and creates a chain reaction that keeps electrons in a perpetual continuous flow or what we may call superconduction. Zero point residuum waves and the superconduction of the human body causes us to have an aura, scientists refer to as the Meisner effect. The Meisner effect is defined as *"the expulsion of a magnetic field from the interior of an organism or material that is in the process of becoming a superconductor, that is losing its resistance to the flow of electrical currents when cooled below a particular temperature, called the transition temperature, which is usually close to absolute zero."* Refer to this the next time you find yourself at a crossroad between light and darkness in you spiritual development. When we bring about balance between forces, we allow for even greater manifestations to reveal themselves.

More On Vibrations

It should be obvious now that everything in our universe is vibration. It is a universal law that everything from the highest frequencies down to the densest forms of matter is essentially vibrational energy. This universal law was taught by our ancestors and has been verified by modern science. The shorter the wavelength is the higher and finer the frequency will be. The longer the wavelength is the lower and denser the frequency will be. We are all responsible for the vibrations that we emit out into the universe and we are just as responsible for the ones that we choose to entertain.

It is said that our world is composed of more space than matter, but we tend to place a higher priority on all the apparently solid things. We also have a misunderstanding when it comes to the nature of "space". The idea of nothing as taught by the western educational system doesn't have a true place in our universe. The truth is that what we assume is empty space, is in actuality magnetism and we are always influencing it and determining how it is expressed from the thoughts we think to the vibrations we make with our physical bodies. Physics tells us that space makes up 99% of what we perceive as reality however the two physics theories of general relativity and quantum theory do not fully agree when it comes to explaining this. Humility and reverence for the works of the ancients is needed more than ever for clarity in these fields and professions.

Each of us vibrates according to the manner in which we think and how we behave. We can look at ourselves like living walking tones that affect everything that we come into contact with and indirectly everything else. Life can be viewed as a huge symphony orchestra with all of the sentient beings and even the inanimate objects playing the role of a musician or an instrument. The tones that we embody and give off can fluctuate depending on how we choose to live and what we allow ourselves to be influenced by. This only reiterates the fact that we are responsible for our own energy and for the effects that we have on others. There is no escaping this fact. Responsibility goes hand in hand with what many call free will.

Higher Vibrations

Higher vibrations from states of consciousness associated with love, gratitude, appreciation, grace, consideration, compassion, etc. cause the heart to beat in a coherent manner which means that its rhythm, frequency, and balance is in harmony with the rest of the body and the surrounding environment. The impressions from these higher states of consciousness impact the human body thru the autonomic nervous system, which is the system that helps us to maintain health and balance by automatically ensuring that all of our bodily functions are working properly and in concert with one another. This system is ran by our subconscious mind so we have the ability to influence it indirectly simply by altering the ways that we think and feel. It is easiest to program the autonomic nervous system when we slow down our brain waves via practices like meditation or various forms of relaxation where we can block out external influences and have our way with our minds. We tend to solely seek answers from all sorts of places external to us when we actually have the ability to change and manipulate neurotransmitters, hormones, genes, proteins, and enzymes from thought alone. Let us keep in mind that the realm of possibilities and potential exist inside of us while the material or physical world simply reflects and reveals those possibilities.

It is important for us to discontinue following trends that may not be in our best interest to practice. We need more personalized approaches because we are all different and our bodies and minds will respond to things according to our specific conditions. When we understand the basics and then the variety of options that Mother Nature provides us with we can create step-by-step plans of action to get us from our undesirable places to where we truly want to be. It should be understood by now that greatest of vibrations for any man or woman can only be attained when he or she is honoring and respecting their divine and exclusive relationship with the absolute. This is achieved at the highest levels when we are fulfilling our purpose here on Earth.

No one knows us better than our cosmic mother. If we expect to move our awareness up and past heart center into the highest of vibrations, we must be honest with ourselves about what is too heavy to carry with us and what no longer serves us. We cannot continue to fool ourselves about our physical, social, or mental attachments.

Ch.31: On Spirit and Matter

What we refer to as physical matter is only a denser form of spirit. It can be described as a form of vibrational energy that occupies space for a given amount of time and has both a mass and weight. The particles that compose matter seem as though they are immobilized and are unable to travel as radiant energy. These apparently immobile particles weave and interact with one another due to the various levels of magnetism produced from the elements composing the said form of matter. This phenomenon is referred to as intermolecular force. The protons involved tend to carry an electric charge while electrons in most cases carry a magnetic charge. The mutual pull from these two particles causes them to bond together in atomic structures called molecules. Molecules then bind together and begin the secondary stages of materialization. We say secondary here because the primal cause occurs much before the denser formations are made. The organization and formation of matter is initially caused by consciousness and the finer versions of spirit.

Matter has four phases or forms and they are as follows: plasma, gas, liquid, solid. The latter is not actually still and immovable as most are led to believe but instead solid forms of matter continue to vibrate like all other things. The difference is that the wavelengths are longer and the movement is so slow that it appears to be motionless. Water is unique in that it can be altered and expresses itself in any of the said states of matter. It can be subtle and gaseous in the form of vapor, liquid in the form of drinking water, plasma in the form of EZ or structured water or apparently solid in the form of ice. We as human beings are distinguished from other forms of creation in some subtle but profound ways. We are beings of light as all things in existence are made up of light. We are watery beings as the human body is basically a water machine and we are also crystal beings as our bodies are composed of many mineral combinations and arrangements.

Ch.32: The Universe Is Mental

"The war is for your mind"

-Dominec Holmes

"Thinking is dielectric in nature and allows one to draw directly from the cosmic clay of the universe. The production of a thought determines the quality and agenda of the magnetic field it produces."

-Asa Lockett

We are in a war right now. We are fighting for both our lives and our minds.

Be mindful of the content you allow into your field of awareness. It is one thing to take note of something and to identify whether it is beneficial or harmful to you. It is another thing to constantly entertain an idea, allowing it to replicate itself and make a bed in your mental space. All thoughts vibrate. It would benefit one to seek out where our thoughts originate in the first place. We can pontificate and preach about it in literature but the real benefit comes when you consider and/or experience the reality of what is being conveyed. Consciousness is essentially all there is and it ranges from its subtle to its denser states. Our self-awareness allows for us to remember who we are as opposed to the things we create. Many of us get caught up in our creations and forget that we are the causers of all things manifested in out lives.

The standard for consciousness is extremely low when it is compared to our true potential as human beings. We were born into a world where the paradigm was designed to strip the energy away from the people. We also ignorantly destroy ourselves from habits and beliefs that cater to our egos instead of our well-being. This is possible because most of us do not have a knowledge of self or of the universe we live in. The end result of this ignorance is what we see today in the world. Dis-ease is rampant and seems to not only be the norm but it is expected eventually because of the nature of our habits and their known consequences. Mental disorders are at an all time high because we were never taught how to think properly. We the people are separated in our beliefs and fragmented in our actions, affecting the world we share collectively and this results in a number of unnecessary conflicts. We can agree to have different objectives without belittling or harming one another when we operate from an altruistic place. It is a known fact among those who have an eye to see that there is actually enough abundance on the planet for everyone to have overflow. When we replace the wars with cooperation we create the potential to see a melting pot of amazing ideas from all over the world ready for use by humanity as a whole.

Strive to bring about balance between your imagination and your external world. Know and understand that every time you think a thought, your mind recalibrates and your relationship with the universe changes. Because the average person thinks the same thoughts day after day, the changes made in their lives are so small and subtle that they can be unnoticeable. Be sure to be active and involved during your meditative states to make undeniable adjustments and understand that it is your responsibility to maintain the vibrations you achieve after your meditation sessions are finished. Identifying the ideas and thoughts you want to manifest is important but consistency and the actions necessary to anchor and materialize those thoughts are just as important. Every thought counts because every thought produces its own ripple or waves for the universe to respond to.

The conscious mind is what you are using to read this book right now.

The Conscious Mind
The conscious mind is abstract
The conscious mind is aware of sensory perception
The conscious mind is analytical
The conscious mind is our reasonable
The conscious mind is where we make decisions
The conscious mind is where we visualize and recall memories
The conscious mind thinks and evaluates
The conscious mind what we use to direct and steer ourselves in life
The conscious mind is what we use to concentrate and to pay attention to things
The conscious mind is masculine in nature

The subconscious mind is where all the magic happens.

The Subconscious Mind
The subconscious mind is always at work
The subconscious mind records every decision and experience that we make
The subconscious mind is influenced the most from symbols
The subconscious mind is molded and altered by repetition
The subconscious mind does not discern between right and wrong or good and bad
The subconscious mind exists in the eternal present moment
The subconscious mind is responsible for approximately 95% of our behavior
The subconscious mind takes everything literally
The subconscious mind is extremely receptive
The subconscious mind is feminine in nature

Thought has been shown to influence the growth of seeds and the mind has been proven capable of bending metals and interacting on both an electrical and mechanical level. A bothered or angry person may experience more computer crashes than a person who is poised emotionally. High vibration thoughts create an alkaline field while lower states of consciousness cause acidity and the weakening in the fields of surrounding organisms.

Neuroplasticity is one of our brain's superpowers. It is the brain's capability to arrange itself and reorganize neural pathways in response to thinking, learning or new experiences.

Neural pathways are made up on neurons connected by dendrites. They are created in the brain based on our decisions, habits, and behaviors. We can alter or redirect them at any given time but especially during meditations while the body is in a relaxed state.

Neurotransmitters are chemical messengers that transmit signals from neurons to cells. They are created every time we produce a thought and serve as a bridge between our consciousness and our body. Some scientists even describe them as being the chemical version of our thoughts.

Neuro Linguistic Programming or *NLP* allows for one to make conscious behavioral changes. It is a way to reprogram the nervous system thru the use of language. An easy way to practice this technique is to make recordings of yourself speaking positively or affirmatively about yourself and then listen to these recordings early in the morning or on repeat as you fall asleep.

Everything vibrates and the brain is no different. Depending on how we think, waves are produced in the brain that correspond to our consciousness. These *brain waves* can be altered at any moment and are responsible for the way that we perceive reality both internally and externally. They are rhythmic or repetitive patterns of neural activity that take place in our central nervous system. They are measured in cycles or the number of times that neurons are firing per second.

Brain Wave State	Hertz	Description
Delta	0.5-4 Hz	Deep sleep
Theta	4-8 Hz	Day dreaming
Alpha	8-12 Hz	The imaginary world
Beta	12-30 Hz	Normal wake state
Gamma	30-100 Hz	Extreme concentration

The mind and its thinking can be viewed as a cosmic hand and a magic wand. From reading up until this point it is easy to see how it is capable of anything. The universe is mental and everything that exist here on the material plane is only mental energy that has slowed down and become materialized. This book was once a thought. Anything that you have ever purchased and any place that you've visited was once an idea is someone's mind. The brain is similar to a radio transmitter in that it constantly receives and sends out thoughts in the form of waves. The brain is also a powerful generator of energy and vibrations. The wavelengths produced by the brain depend on the mental development of the individual. This means that it may be difficult for a person with long and slow mental waves to understand someone with high and short mental waves. We are all at our respective levels when it comes to our mental growth and development.

Any and everything that can be imagined in the mind can be accomplished in the material world. The mind is more powerful and influential than we typically make it out to be. In order for us to achieve greater states of health we must eventually improve the condition of our minds and of those around us. It is also important for us to remain mindful of the quality of people that we surround ourselves with and spend the most time around. Since all meetings and conversations result in an exchange of magnetism and mental substance it is critical for us to pay attention to whether or not people make us feel better or worse after interacting with them as it is a sign of how they have affected us and how are body and mind responds to them.

The majority of people randomly jump from one thought to another as they are influenced and altered by circumstances and external sources. This leads to them having a scattered mind and they end up wasting unnecessary amounts of energy. By remaining present and becoming intentional with our thinking we can better preserve our energy and determine the outcome of our personal magnetic fields so that our vibrations are used to manifest more desired results. This should not be expected to occur over night. Practice and consistency will prove to be beneficial and essential for this mental accomplishment. It must also be understood that all disease begins in the mind and eventually manifest in the body if the mental imbalance is not addressed or if the poor habits are continuously performed.

Section 6 Summary

Our oppressors have done the absolute most to eliminate the light from melanated people in this world. Our land was stolen, our people were taken captive, our land was stolen, and our rich histories were stripped away from us. Black people are the original people of this planet. We seeded this planet. We were chosen from above to teach science, and law and order. However, societies do not recognize what we've done.

Truth is, black is powerful, and Asa has shown us how powerful it is from a physical, metaphysical, and spiritual standpoint. The void is where everything we know originates. Again, the original man and woman on this planet were black people and they seeded this entire world. Today, black culture is popular culture. We are lit! We are powerful. The moment we embrace that reality as a people, there's nothing that can be done against us. Most importantly, once we walk in our divinity, we will be able to heal ourselves in all aspects. We will be able to break the chains of spiritual, mental, and physical bondage and be the Gods and Goddesses on earth like we were designed to be. We will be walking examples of optimal health like we were on the motherland ages ago. We can be that right in Urban America. Black Is Powerful.

Regarding the color spectrum, I strongly recommend studying chakras which are subtle energy centers in our bodies which channel physical and mental balance in us. Each chakra corresponds with a color on the spectrum, from the heaviest color red to the lightest violet. Understanding concepts like chakras will better equip you to understand everything described in this section.

The Habits

Ch.33: On Meditation

If you are interest in making your brain larger and stronger, you should consider meditating. Scientific research from both Harvard University and MIT on people who meditate reveals that it caused their brains to grow significantly larger in areas responsible for learning, memory, concentration and control of emotions. People who meditate have also been shown to have increased brain connectivity and thickness when compared to those who do not meditate at all. Research shows that the longer a person meditates the larger their brain becomes and the more capable it is us functioning at greater levels. Meditation has also been proven to increase one's level of intelligence, creativity and their sense of intuitive perception. Fresh air is important when striving to replicate these improvements in your personal life since oxygenation of the brain is vital to its performance. Just as plants need the purest air possible in order to grow to their strongest state and reach their greatest potential, so do our brains in order to develop into their most profound states as well. You can find this air in forests, mountains, coastlines, and wherever trees and greenery are most abundant. If you live in a city and your environment is devoid of these oxygen producers then your air is likely to be low in oxygen and lacking vitality and high energy levels. Purchasing plants to beautify and liven your home can help but does not substitute for what nature offers. Also complete breathing will benefit all who make it a practice to full up the lungs by inhaling and sending oxygen to the lower regions of the diaphragm as opposed to heavy short breaths directed at the top of the chest that only feel up a portion of the lungs. This practice strengthens the lungs in the same way that weight lifting builds ones muscles.

Ch.34: Healthy Habits

We need to be more aware of our habits and the effects that they have on us. When we create habits we are creating rituals. This is why we should become more mindful of those things that we find ourselves doing repeatedly and consciously choose those specific things we wish to see manifested in our lives. Repetition is a formula for instant results. Choice is Magnetic in nature and the repeating of a particular choice only strengthens its magnetism. Our habits put us into the conditions we find ourselves in. The condition we are in determines the direction we are facing in life.

Recommended Habits
Genuinely listen as opposed to simply hearing what someone is saying
Begin your days with gratitude
Plan ahead and do so with planetary energies in mind
Practice to make improvements
Be consistent with beneficial practices
Remain hydrated daily
Eat to prepare you for the activities you have ahead of you
Think before you speak and act
Live in the moment as opposed to dwelling on the past or worrying about the future
Center yourself often throughout the day

Habits that are in alignment with our life's purpose tend to reward us with a pleasant shift in attitude. When we change our innermost attitudes, we change our relationship with the universe both in and outside of us. The innermost attitudes we choose to carry throughout our days impregnate all of the choices we make and the activities we involve ourselves in. Our environments and the people we choose to interact with are affected by our innermost attitudes as well.

Recommended Morning Habits or Routine
Wake up to gratitude
Drink a glass of water with lemon or lime
Meditate in order to determine the trajectory of your day
Review your daily agenda and visualize yourself accomplishing each task
Exercise for about 15 minutes to get your blood flowing for the day ahead of you

Recommended Evening Habits or Routine
Reflect on the way your day went and find ways that you can change for the better
Read for 30 minutes to feed your mind content ideal manifesting the best you
Drink a cup of non caffeinated tea
Plan out and imagine how you want your next day to go
Meditate to create the neural pathways necessary for your personal success

Diseases are less hereditary than bad habits. We tend to mimic our family members and those we spend the most time around or observing. Be sure to take the time to sift thru those things that you find yourself doing repeatedly in order to ensure that you are not contributing to your own detriment.

Ch.35: Getting Back To Our Center

The center point is the opposite of all things. When we pull attention back into ourselves and away from the world of external phenomena, we have the opportunity to wield and change our internal condition, which results in a corresponding adjustment in the way we have to deal with things outside of us. The external world, even though it may appear to be the same, by law deals with and becomes affected by the inward changes that we have made to ourselves. The unmanifest is the precursor to what we know of as cause and effect and serves as a cosmic womb in a way for both to exist in. when we find ourselves getting caught up in life's web of events, we can always count on our ability to go within and become something greater. Remember that all of the events and circumstances that we find ourselves in are put there on purpose by the universe in order to teach us or remind us of whatever it is we need to be taught or reminded of in that moment. When we are hardheaded, the events will seem to be reoccurring but when we take the time to look, listen, and observe what the universe is showing us, we can grasp what is being conveyed and move on to the next level of growth and development. Becoming and remaining centered doesn't just allow for us to see things clearly. It keeps us from straying too far off balance signaling to Mother Nature that we are in need of yet another lesson. When we are centered we can tap into our true latent powers instead of being limited by acting from ego, thinking from places that are opinionated and not from our source where there is a natural sense of knowing. We pretty much run into trouble every time we place our attention in places too far from our core for long periods of time. It is important to know that this state of centeredness takes us beyond the mind, as we know it. Think of the mind as a medium in this world that bridges our spiritual activities and our external manifestations. Meditation is an excellent way to get better at balancing ourselves so that we can do better at remembering who we truly are rather than whom we tend to be. Whatever we choose to do ultimately is up to us but know that the universe is always responding to whatever we end up choosing. We can observe all the options we want but choice is magnetic by nature. When attempting to center self, it may take time to get it down pact at first but it is more than worth it because it will affect every other part of our life. It will also make the healing process easier to get thru. You are the dot in the middle of the circle and the circle is a reflection of what you choose to do at your center. Don't overthink it and make it more complicated than it is. Remember Mother Nature is plain and simplified as it gets. Out of all our teachers in life, she is hands down the easiest to learn from. To be centered is a cosmological and sacred geometrical experience.

Section 7 Summary

The healthy habits described above achieve one thing – Staying centered. Power starts with balance. When you are centered, nothing can defeat you. When you are centered, you can achieve anything. Your body is naturally engineered to understand what its center is. For example, Shaolin Kenpo 1st Degree Dan Keith Horton of Detroit, Michigan proves to his students that humans automatically know their center by instructing them to pick an ink pen up off the ground, which is placed at a slight distance, without moving their feet. Every student I've witnessed perform this exercise does it the same way. Students will carefully lower their bodies, place one hand on the ground, while reaching out to grab the ink pen. No one falls over and no one moves their feet. When performing the exercise, students just know what to do.

Our bodies have been calibrated to find its center to draw power to do whatever it wants to do. Being from and living in Urban America, especially as a poor minority, there are many weapons formed against us to take us away from our center – people from my neighborhood have the saying that someone or something has "knocked me off my square." Being knocked off your square sends a ripple effect throughout your physical, quantum, and metaphysical worlds. Despite this, we are the only ones to blame when we lose control of our center. We cannot control the actions of others or the circumstances that come to us sometimes, but we can always control how we feel about them and most importantly how to act on them. Staying centered equips you with the control of your spirit and mind which will positively affect your body and its physical abilities.

The healthy habits described in this section barely described anything physical. In fact, more of the exercises required you to be still, like meditation and reflection. Every day, we confuse strength with power. They are indeed two totally different concepts. Strength requires physical exercises that build muscle. Nothing wrong with that. But strength is rooted in power, which is your mind-crafted will, determination, and painter of your reality. We need powerful men and women in our community to bring about a healthier hood and that power will come from the spirit and mind. The body will always follow.

Elementary School

Section 8 Intro

Instead of summarizing this section, I will simply introduce it as the section that shows us that our bodies are made up of everything found in the universe which reinforces the truth that we are connected to everything. What Asa is teaching us below are all the ingredients used to create life on this planet and beyond. Our bodies are made of hundreds of millions of many particles which is a small reflection of the universe which is made of a gazillion particles. Again, we are connected to everything in this universe. We are a vessel which holds some of everything in this universe. What a beautiful thing!

Ch.36: Elementary School

On Ether

Ether or Aether is the fundamental substance that precedes the four basic elements that we are all familiar with today. Another simplified way of describing it is to say that it is pure potentiality. Its attribute is the same as what we refer to as infinity or the absolute. This is also a more modern term for what our ancestors called the waters of nu or nun. Nikola Tesla even said, *"Light is a longitudinal disturbance in the Ether"*. According to the Rosicrucian Fellowship and other secret societies preserving some of the ancient wisdom of our ancestors, there are four types of ethers that serve as a foundation to each of the four basic elements.

Matter is made manifest to us in the continual interplay between fire, air, water, and earth.

Each element has two specific characteristics. There is one main one and there is another that serves as a connecting medium to the other elements. For example, fire is hot and dry and Earth is dry and cold. Water is cold and wet (moist) while air is moist and hot. Inside the human body we can assign the earth element to bones and nerves, the water element to the lymphatic system, the air element to the respiratory system, and the fire element to the pulsating of warm blood throughout the entirety of the body. The same forces found in nature are found inside of us.

On Fire

Notice that when human beings die, they stop giving off heat. The fire inside of us is the life force energy that permeates and fuels the human body. This vitalizing energy is carried throughout the body by the blood as it removes waste and delivers nutrients to our cells. Remember that iron (ruled by Mars) is at the core of the blood as it magnetizes the plethora of elements our bodies are composed of. The fiery exciting energy here serves as the ordering principle, which determines how the remaining elemental forces will be influenced. Most people seem to have a problem with accepting the fact that the universe is alive and naturally intelligent. We all have the ability to use introspection at any given time to bare witness to this. The same power and supremacy causing the planets to move exists inside of us and causes our very heart to beat. We tend to associate subtle with weak instead of acknowledging how influential and impactful something like fire can be. It is the active representation and expressed arrangement of the ethers, which are antecedent to it. Fire in its extreme forms consumes anything its path and transforms it. It is difficult to control and is both combustive and impulsive. When fire able to slow down, it interacts instead of overpowering, which allows for a more balanced transformation to take place. Physiologically fire manifests as a fever, which purifies or burns off pathogens and toxins that pose a threat to the body.

(Upward active motion i.e. smoke rises)

The Element of Fire
Intense
Passionate
Electrifying
Inspirational
Insightful

On Air

It is invisible yet it is vital to and responsible for the functioning and preservation of sentient beings. We are all familiar with the fact that we can go days and weeks possibly without water and food but only minutes if not seconds without fresh air. While it is comprised of various gases, the oxygen in it is essential to our breathing and a number of biological events that go unnoticed by the average unstudied person. Just as a flame needs oxygen to continue to burn, our thinking and brain functioning is dependent on the quality of air that we breathe in. Mother Nature has blessed us with a priceless reciprocal relationship with the plants as they utilize our exhaled carbon dioxide while we inhale the fresh oxygen that they release. A lack of fresh oxygen to the brain increases oxidative stress and can harm or kill the brain cells. The elements work in concert together and we can see this easily when we observe the affinity that oxygen has for the iron in our body. Air in general has a magnetic nature to it. Notice how the birds base their movements off the magnetic currents flowing through the sky and are able to interpret the weather days and sometimes weeks before humans even become aware of certain phenomena. Air is also associated with the mind and all things mental so you may notice different schools of thought teaching about different breathing practices used to induce different brain wave states. Even though air is not visible to the naked eye, its role is just as significant as any other element as they are all expressions of the same underlying universal substance. Even though air is not visible, in its extreme forms like tornados and hurricanes, it can decimate an entire community. It is impossible to pin down and it prefers to circulate. It can however be calmed and settled down and this attribute can be an excellent teacher to us as it reminds us of the importance and power of being present and poised. The air element can be useful in healing as we use it to uplift our energy when our emotions are too heavy or when the body becomes to stagnant, lacking circulation and movement. It serves us when we honor and respect it by refreshing us after breathing in deep or complete breaths.

(Significant invisible activities and levity i.e. air lifts)

The Element of Air
Current
Permeability
Refreshing
Catalyzing

On Water

Water is extremely underestimated in the world today yet it is responsible for the possibility and success of most things that we benefit from. It maintains life in humans, plants, and animals. Water cleanses out toxins from the body and delivers them over to the liver and kidneys for disposal. It lubricates the intestines and helps to prevent constipation and other digestive set backs. Water has been proven time after time to assist in all of our biological functions. It is feminine in nature and extremely receptive however it is powerful enough to sink a ship or breakdown the toughest of materials over time. Had it not been for the water element, none of us would have been developed in our mother's womb. It clears, nurtures, and sustains all that it comes into contact with and this includes diseases and substances that we know to be harmful.

The shape and the quality of the water in our body plays a vital role in determining how it will express itself and function. We will speak further on this in a moment. Water is soaked into the earth and assumes the shape of its environment. We also witness the process of bonding as it reassembles itself to substances that allow for it. Physiologically, water nourishes us while supporting neurological and overall biological processes. It helps us to conduct and store bioavailable energy in the form of electricity. The water molecule is the antenna of all life in the universe.

The human body consists of 99.999% water. This water is changed and conditioned by the choices we make daily. A dehydrated person may experience a sluggish and weak body while a truly healthy person may feel charged up and fully capable at any given moment. The difference is in the condition of the waters in the body. Vibration has a significant impact here as well. The innermost attitude of a person is just as if not more important than the condition of the physical body that they exist in. Highly structured water also known as H3O2 has special properties and is described as living water. Its negative charge allows it to hold energy exactly like a battery. The water contained in fresh fruits and vegetables is already in this structured form.

More on Water

When it comes to water and its properties, there are a number of doctors and scientists who have contributed to our most advanced levels of understanding when it comes to this element but here we would like to highlight one who made significant contributions through their experimentation. Dr. Masaru Emoto has provided us with fascinating examples of how water behaves on a microscopic level and these findings allow for us to make better decisions in regards to our relationship with water and its impact on our health. He was born on July 22, 1943 in Yokohama, Japan. He graduated from Yokohama Municipal University and continued studies at the Open International University. Shortly after receiving his Doctorate of Alternative Medicine, he was introduced to the concept of micro cluster water and Magnetic Resonance Analysis technology, which sparked his fascination with water and its mysterious properties. He went on to author several best selling books, including *Messages from Water* and *The Hidden Messages in Water* which contain photographs of ice crystals and how they alter in form in response to surrounding energy and vibrations. His pictures revealed that when water is exposed to high vibrations via positive thoughts, beautiful music, meditations or sincere prayers, the crystals appear in beautifully symmetrical shapes resembling a six pointed star like what you would see in a snowflake. When water is exposed to low vibrations like hatred, anger, fear, negative thinking, chaotic music like heavy metal, or ridicule, the water takes on sloppy looking shapes resembling mud or disorderliness.

Dr. Emoto's goal was to get the world to understand that consciousness contributes to the healing process in a very significant way. If our bodies are composed of majority water, one can easily imagine what occurs inside of us on a regular bases as we continuously fluctuate between moods and modes of thought. It would be wise of us to apply this simple but life altering break through to our daily considerations and to make it habit of operating at higher levels in order to bypass the health hazards caused by low vibrational choices. To make this plainer one can say that the higher vibrations promote a balanced state of alkalinity within the body as opposed to low vibrations, which will result in an unbalanced state of acidity and a weakened immune system.

The two-time Nobel Prize winner Linus Pauling is credited with being the first to introduce the theory of water memory transfer. His contributions to science point to the idea that the state of the water molecules affects brain function and that like Dr. Emoto, vibrations and resonance affect the formation of water molecules.

(Feminine and extremely powerful i.e. capable of breaking down any substance to its basic constituents)

The Element of Water
Fluid
Adaptable
Flowing
Flexible
Emotional

*To pay homage to the ancestor responsible for pioneering our modern day understanding of the importance of water and its divine features, seek out and study the works of the great aquatologist Dr. Mona Harrison.

On Earth

The Earth is a huge magnet and everything, even an ocean, is governed by magnetism and the pull of ions.

Earth provides us with stability and serves as the perfect foundation for building and constructing on the physical plane. While it is composed of many different parts, its key element is carbon, which is the most cohesive element on our periodic table. The key word for the earth is pragmatism. Physiologically, the earth element sustains us thru its food and the metabolic processes. It also provides us with safety, security, and dependability. Earth is a living, self-organizing, and self-regulating system. Earth has also been shown to control its own temperature and conditions.

The Earth is exposed to certain radiation belts due to the unique movement of our solar system. Celestial radiation affects our biological systems significantly. Sunshine, sunspots, solstices, equinoxes, both solar and lunar eclipses, and the daily and monthly cycles of the moon affect the tides and activities of ions in the atmosphere. Minerals, hormones, and other phytochemicals in human, plant, and animal life are changed by the Earth's magnetic field and these radiations that permeate throughout our universe.

The Earth's magnetic field and its currents flows both north and south. This geomagnetic energy pulses or vibrates at 7.83 Hertz. Studies indicate that in areas where currants of geomagnetic energy are intense, people grow stronger and are healthier. This is another reason why those of us living in cities and urban areas further from the equator should become more proactive when it comes to our physical health. Where the earth's magnetic energy is softer or less concentrated, people tend to suffer greater rates of debilitating disorders.

(Downward and receptive i.e. plants grow roots deep into the earth)

The Element of Earth
Repository
Grounding
Texture
Apparently Solid
Material
Vehicle
Container
Physical
Stage

None of these basic elements or expressions from nature are superior to the others. Each one balances out its opposite and harmonizes with the remaining two. Also, it must be understood that when it comes to maintaining health, all four of these elements need to remain in equilibrium because without balance, true health is not attainable. These basic elements are used as a way to understand the world around us and have been expressed in some form or another on every continent for thousands of years. Even though they can serve as categories for it, these four forces should not be confused with what we refer to as the periodic table of elements.

Our ancestors honored and respected the elements to the degree that they associated deific names to many of them. As with most things, Europeans claim to have discovered the elements on the so called periodic table but our ancestors were much more advanced in their knowledge and understanding of the universe. Walls, pillars, and monuments have been uncovered reveling our awareness of the substances making up our universe. Every so-called element on the periodic table is a combination and/or arrangement of hydrogen. It is the expression of the most primal material in our universe and is unparalleled when it comes to energy production. The bulk of the energy our body produces comes from basic chemical and physical processes. They yield much more energy than other sources do through nuclear reactions. Elements are formed by fusion and work together to build more complex versions of creation. Fusion is the name of the process that powers the Sun and other stars as hydrogen atoms merge to create different forms of matter. Fission is defined as the action of dividing or splitting something into multiple parts. Both fusion and fission are physical processes that produce massive amounts of energy. The forces latent within Mother Nature use these processes to guide the arrangement of the elements and cause for them to follow specific patterns. This is also one of the first expressions of what we refer to as sacred geometry.

An element is a substance that cannot be broken down any further. The minerals and vitamins differ in their ratio of elements and how the elements are joined together through ionic or covalent bonding. Minerals are inorganic substances required by our body in various amounts to complete its everyday functions. Vitamins are slightly more complex and are made up of minerals and finer elements like hydrogen and oxygen. Minerals help to sustain and stabilize the body while vitamins energize and vitalize us. Elements have three types of actions in us. They are known to relate to each other in different ways resulting in synthesizing, decomposition, or displacement. When the elements relate to each other in harmony and balance we say that they synergize. Decomposition is when organic substances break down into simpler organic or inorganic forms of matter like carbon dioxide, water, and sugars. When elements relate to each other by substituting, redirecting actions, or move away from each other while retaining a non-polar relationship it is referred to as displacement. El in some ancient languages means "god" or "light" so the word element even though it may have its westernized definition can thought of as a substance made out of light (hydrogen) to be used by a child of god, an entity or a sentient being.

The combination of elements provides a code that determines all aspects of our form.

Ch.37: Inside of You

Minerals Are Crystals

Crystals are a record of the force that produced them, thus their shapes and all their other attributes. Here we see the law of correspondence displayed clearly. Denser forms of matter are only the temporary arrangements of pure potential. The variation of form is determined by the relative arrangement or variation of the potential energy. A simple way of saying this is crystals are a storehouse for frequency and vibration. They are uniquely condensed forms and arrangements of light. They can be categorized by their characteristics and the effects that they have in our bodies or the way that they express themselves when interacting with other portions of Mother Nature. Minerals are crystals.

Sacred geometry is mathematically sound and reveals a profound order in all things, especially in the codes that are responsible for the creation of life. Shape denotes function in our universe. Our hands are composed of fingers, a thumb, a surface and a palm so that we can grip. Our eyes are designed a particular way giving us the ability to utilize light in order to perceive the world around us. On a smaller level food is composed of certain minerals and complexes that perform a definite way inside of us. Those who practice the craft of masonry know and understand the significance and importance of geometry.

Calcium is an essential mineral that serves as the primary building block for skeletal and dental structures in the body. It is necessary for proper fetal growth and formation. Calcium also soothes the nervous system.

Carbon is an essential mineral that serves as the building block for of organic matter. Carbon is the primary organizing mineral in all organic materials. It is the most cohesive element in the universe.

Chlorine is an essential mineral best known for its cleansing properties as it expels wastes and impurities from the body. It is both germicidal and anti-bacterial. Chlorine is a key element in the digestive process and when combined with hydrogen, they form hydrochloric acid which is the necessary digestive secretion found in the stomach. It also has pain-reducing properties.

Chromium is the trace mineral responsible for proper insulin and glucose balance in the blood and also proper functioning of the spleen and pancreas.

Copper is a trace mineral and is found in all bodily tissues. It is a key element of the amino acid tyrosine, which is a major building block of melanin. Copper partners up with iron for hemoglobin production and is necessary for the body to be able to conduct ionic energy.

Fluorine fortifies the human body and reinforces all hard tissues like bones, teeth, ligaments, sinus, nails, etc. It is acts like an anti-oxidant and prevents the decay of these tissues. Fluorine also has germicidal and disinfecting qualities.

Hydrogen is the most basic element and is essentially what all others are comprised of. It means, "to produce water" and it serves as the moisturizing element in the body. All living organism contain hydrogen, as it is the medium in which all cellular activity takes place. It is present in almost all biological processes.

Iron is the most magnetic element in our solar system. It is an essential mineral found at the core of our blood. Iron has an affinity with oxygen and serves as the means by which we attract it into our body. Many physical ailments are caused from the body being deficient in this mineral while on the other hand, an abundance of iron results in radiance and vitality.

Lithium is a trace mineral, which the body requires in small amounts for mental stability. Lithium is beneficial when treating depression and many different types of substance abuse.

Magnesium is an essential mineral that has been found to be both relaxing and nourishing to the nervous system. It is vital to optimal brain function and promotes peaceful sleep. Magnesium alkalizes the body, cools down fevers, reduces inflammation, and sharpens perception.

Manganese is an essential mineral that improves both memory and alertness. It also helps to boost mind and body coordination. Manganese balances bile activity, harmonizes the nervous system, and increases resistance/immune response. It relieves edginess and anxiety, and increases the capacity for one to experience higher vibration emotions.

Nitrogen is yet another key element found in organic chemistry. It is a base component of amino acids and melanin compounds. It is located in the flesh, tissues, bodily fluids, hair, skin, nails, eyes and connective tissues. It is the element responsible for holding and fastening the body and its parts together.

Oxygen is the volatile and active element in biochemistry. It means "to produce acid" and is essential to health as every cell requires it in order to remain vital. Cancer cells cannot exist in a fully oxygenated cell. It helps with the assimilation of nutrients, promotes cell regeneration, strengthens mental activities, and helps the body to maintain a youthful appearance.

Phosphorus means, "light bearer" and lives out its name as it has the ability to radiate light. Inside the human body, phosphorus is the element the brain uses to think, memorize, visualize, and reason. It is improves sexual function and is essential for reproduction. Phosphorus can also be found in muscles tissues as well as our bone structure.

Potassium is an alkalizing element and is necessary for maintaining a healthy ph balance in the body. It neutralizes acidic conditions, alkalizes the bloodstream, and increases the overall efficiency of the body's systems. Potassium eliminates waste from the cells, improves the body's capacity to heal, and prevents health challenges. It is essential for proper circulation and nerve functioning.

Selenium is a trace mineral that is necessary for the body to maintain its elasticity. Selenium allows for the body to grow and mature properly and is needed for fertility in both women and men.

Silica plays a vital role in the nervous system as it facilitates the transmission of neural impulses. It is considered to be a magnetic element and it crucial for neural impulses to jump from neuron to neuron. Silica is also a building block for hair, bone, teeth, skin, and nails. It allows these structures to maintain a firm yet elastic feature.

Sodium is also an alkalizing element and it helps with insuring that the lymphatic system and bloodstream remain charged. Sodium is stored in the stomach and is the element that neutralizes acids. It is necessary for proper digestion and has the ability to attract and to house water. Sodium is also an ion carrier qualifying it as an electrolyte in our body's fluids.

Sulfur is one of the elements found in certain types of melanin and is the basis of the amino acid cysteine. It is vital for regulating body temperature and also the body's ability to produce and retain heat.

Zinc is a trace mineral and is very crucial to performance of the body. DNA synthesis and replication is dependent upon sufficient amounts of zinc. It is instrumental to the health of the reproductive system and plays a critical role in restoration from burns, cuts, and minor injuries. Many enzymes that play a role in digestion and respiration contain zinc.

Minerals	Recommended Daily Dosages
Calcium	1,500 mcg
Chromium	150 mcg
Copper	3 mg
Iron	225 mcg
Iodine	18 mg
Magnesium	750 mg
Manganese	2 mg
Molybdenum	30 mcg
Potassium	99 mg
Selenium	200 mcg
Zinc	30mg

Vitamins Are Made Up of Minerals

Vitamins are made up of minerals and more basic substances that work in concert to perform a particular duty in our body. They are necessary for normal cell functioning, growth, and development. A lack of vitamins will result in a lack of vitality in the area of the body that those particular vitamins are responsible for or whatever roles the vitamins are depended on for may be done insufficiently.

Vitamin A in its multiple forms has been shown to prevent night blindness and many other eye issues. It supports healthy skin and can be used as an aid in acne prevention. Vitamin A improves immunity in the body and helps to heal and prevent gastrointestinal ulcers. It protects against cellular pollution, cancer formation, and is needed for skin regeneration. It also assists in the formation of bones and teeth and aids in fat storage. Vitamin A protects our bodies from colds, influenza, and infections. Foods containing beta-carotene are converted to Vitamin A in the liver.

Beta-carotene is an inorganic reddish or orange colored pigment found in fungi, plants, and fruits. It is a precursor to Vitamin A.

Vitamin B1 also known as Thiamine improves circulation and helps with the production of hydrochloric acid. It is also significant in both blood formation and carbohydrate metabolism. Thiamine affects growth disorders, our capacity to learn, and is used for muscle tone in the intestinal walls, the stomach, and the heart.

Vitamin B2 also known as Riboflavin is essential for red blood formation, antibody production, cellular respiration, and growth in general. It helps to alleviate all types of fatigue and is important in the prevention and treatment of eye issues like cataracts. It helps with the metabolism of carbohydrates, fats, and proteins. And when used in combination with vitamin A, it maintains and improves muscles membranes in the gastrointestinal tract. Riboflavin also facilitates the use of oxygen in the body tissues of both the skin and hair. It can assists with the elimination of dandruff and assists with the uptake of Iron and B6 into the body.

Vitamin B3 also known as Niacin is necessary for proper circulation and healthy skin. Vitamin B3 in its niacin form aids in the function of the nervous system and the metabolism of carbohydrates, fats, and proteins. It also assists with the production of hydrochloric acid in the digestive system. It helps to lower cholesterol and is effective in the treatment of schizophrenia and other mental diseases.

Vitamin B5 also known as Pantothenic Acid is referred to as the anti stress vitamin. It plays a significant role in the production of adrenaline, in helping to reduce inflammation, and in the production of antibodies. It also helps with overall vitamin utilization in the body. Pantothenic acid or vitamin B5 helps to convert fats, carbohydrates, and proteins into energy. It is required by all the cells of the body and is concentrated in the organs. It is necessary for normal function of the digestive system and can be beneficial when treating anxiety and depression.

Vitamin B6 also known as Pyridoxine is involved in more bodily functions than any other nutrient. It has affects on our mental and physical states of health. It has proven to be beneficial for individuals suffering from water retention. It is necessary in the production of hydrochloric acid and the absorption of fats and proteins. It also plays a role in the balancing of sodium and potassium balance in the body and helps to promote red blood cell formation.

Vitamin B12 also known as Cyanocobalamin aids in cellular longevity and is required for proper digestive tract functioning, the absorption of nutrients from food, protein synthesis, and the metabolism of both carbohydrates and fats in the body. It helps to prevent nerve damage, maintains virility, and promotes normal growth and development. A lack of vitamin B12 has been associated with the transitioning from the standard American diet into veganism. Chlorella and sea vegetables can be used instead of meat to serve as a quality source of vitamin B12.

The Vitamin B-Complex or the combination of B vitamins helps to maintain the body's nerves, skin, eyes, hair, liver, mouth, and muscle tone in the digestive tract. B Complex vitamins act as coenzymes as they are involved in energy production and may be useful for both anxiety and depression. The B vitamins perform better in the body when used collectively.

Bioflavonoids also known as vitamin P enhance the absorption of Vitamin C and help to relieve the pain from bumps and bruises. They work in harmony with Vitamin c to protect and preserve the structure of capillary blood vessels and promote healthy circulation. They also assist with bowel production and the lowering of cholesterol levels.

Vitamin B7 also known as Biotin assists with cellular growth, fatty acid production, the metabolism of both carbohydrates and proteins, and the utilization of B vitamins. It is needed for healthy hair and skin, thus the constant addition in shampoos and nail related products. Biotin also helps with the production of health sweat glands, muscle tissue and bone marrow.

Vitamin C is an antioxidant necessary for tissue growth and repair making it extremely significant to our muscular system. It is essential to adrenal gland function and healthy gums. Vitamin C protects against the harmful effects caused by pollution, cancer and infection, and improves immunity in the body. It assists in the reduction of cholesterol levels and high blood pressure.

And helps to fix problems like atherosclerosis. Vitamin C is essential in the formation of collagen and helps to protect against blood clotting. It also promotes healing and plays a key role in the production of anti-stress hormones. Depending on a person's health and their environmental location, Vitamin C can be produced in small amounts in our adrenal glands.

Choline is necessary for gall bladder regulation, nerve transmission, liver functioning, and lecithin formation. It reduces excess fat in the liver, aids in hormone production, and is essential in fat and cholesterol metabolism. It can also be used for different disorders of the nervous system.

Vitamin D is required for calcium and phosphorous absorption and utilization. Generally it is essential for growth but especially in the normal growth and development of teeth and bones in children. The vitamin D that we get from food or supplements is meant to serve as a re-activator. Sunlight can be converted directly into vitamin D is ultimately the best source. By allowing ourselves at least an hour or so of sunlight per day we will benefit greatly and meet our daily requirement for vitamin D production.

Vitamin E is an antioxidant and helps to prevent cancer and cardiovascular disease when complimented by the proper levels of mental health. It improves circulation, helps with tissue repair, and is beneficial in treating both fibrocystic breast and premenstrual syndrome. Vitamin E promotes normal clotting and healing by reducing scarring from all sorts of cuts and wounds. It helps to reduce blood pressure, helps to correct cataracts in the eyes, improves overall athletic performance, and assists in easing leg cramps. Vitamin E also helps us to prevent cellular damage and retards the aging process.

Vitamin K is necessary for blood clotting and may also help to prevent osteoporosis. It converts glucose into glycogen for storage in our liver. Only small amounts are needed in order to fulfill its bodily responsibilities.

Vitamin F or unsaturated fatty acids are necessary for normal body function but especially in the areas of the brain and the heart.

Folic acid helps the body with the production of red blood cells and the prevention of changes in the DNA that may lead to cancer formation.

Inositol plays a vital role for hair growth and prevents the hardening of arteries. It is important for lecithin formation and helps to remove excess fat from the liver.

Hesperidin is typically used for blood vessel conditions like hemorrhoids, varicose veins and poor circulation.

Rutin helps to enhance the effects of vitamin C and helps with the treatment of allergies, viruses, arthritis and many other inflammatory diseases.

Para-amino Benzoic Acid also known as PABA is one of the basic components of folic acid and assists with the utilization of pantothenic acid. PABA helps protect against skin cancers and acts as a co-enzyme. They also help with the breakdown of protein and in the formation of red blood cells.

Vitamins	Recommended Daily Dosages
Vitamin A	10,000 IU
Beta-carotene	15,000 IU
Vitamin B1 (Thiamine)	50 mg
Vitamin B2 (Riboflavin)	50 mg
Vitamin B3 (As Niacin)	100 mg
Vitamin B3 (As Niacinamide)	100 mg
Vitamin B6 (Pyridoxine)	50 mg
Vitamin B12 (Cyanocobalamin)	300 mcg
Bioflavonoids	500 mg
Biotin	300 mcg
Vitamin C (with ascorbates)	3,000 mg
Choline	100 mg
Vitamin D	400 IU
Vitamin E	600 IU
Vitamin K	100 mcg
Vitamin F (unsaturated fatty acids)	2,000 mcg
Folic Acid	400 mcg
Inositol	100 mg
Hesperidin	100 mg
Rutin	25 mg
Para-amino Benzoic Acid (PABA)	25 mg

(These mineral and vitamin charts are from the works of Dr. Jewel Pookrum and her colleagues. She is a profound medical doctor and neurosurgeon who studies cater to the melanin dominant people on the planet. Follow this chart

as opposed to using random amounts recommended by companies who cater to the general public or the western standard of health which is typically based on the anatomy and physiology of European males.)

Glycogen is the principle carbohydrate store d in our body. Consuming fruits, vegetables, nuts, and seeds allows for us to partake in antioxidants and whole food mineral/vitamin complexes.

Glands and Hormones

The glands in our body help us to acclimate to our environments and they affect almost every process in the body including metabolism, growth and development, blood pressure levels, sleep cycles, fertility, sexual function, emotions and moods. Essentially they help us to maintain balance or homeostasis in the body. Our glands are the physical counterparts to what metaphysicians and mystics refer to as the chakras. These are said to be energy centers in the body that run up and down our spinal column from the pelvic floor up to the brain. There are many who denounce the existence of chakras, however all students of physics and vibration know and understand that the different glands in us have their individual functions that work together harmoniously. The glands have their specific functions and the law of correspondence ensures us that they also have their specific energetic characteristics to compliment them. The ancients documented these energy centers and today many people use them as a means to navigate internally in order to alter their consciousness where needed in meditations. The hormones secreted from these glands can be stunted or amplified according to the states of consciousness that we choose to entertain and carry around inside of us.

Major Glands	Popular Hormones
Ovaries	Estrogen and Progesterone
Testes	Testosterone
Adrenals	Androgens
Pancreas	Glucagon and Insulin
Thymus	Thymosin
Thyroid and Parathyroids	Thyroxin
Pineal	Serotonin and Melatonin
Pituitary and Hypothalamus	Endorphins and other major hormones

Dehydraepiendestrone or DHEA is a precursor hormone with which other hormones are made. It is essential for mobilization of mineral reserves and managing inflammation throughout the body.

Hormone Pathway
1. Glands detect something needs to change in our body
2. Glands secrete the necessary hormone
3. Hormone travels through the bloodstream
4. Hormone reaches target tissue
5. Change occurs in the body

Each gland creates a specific set of hormones. The gland is stimulated whenever these hormones are needed in the body. Glands can be stimulated in a variety of ways. A change in blood chemistry or different nerve pulsations may instruct a gland to respond in the best manner possible to help the body adjust to new circumstances. The gland releases the hormone into the bloodstream where it travels throughout the body. By way of magnetism the hormone eventually finds its target tissue where it elicits a certain response, like excitement, hunger, arousal or sleepiness.

Ch.38: Hormones, Health, and Emotions

Emotions like calmness, happiness, fear and sadness all affect our alkaline/acid balance.

Hormones also play a major role on the way that we feel throughout the day. They influence our emotions, which makes then indirectly influence every physiological system in the human body. Sweetness in disposition overstimulates the pancreas function, which is alkaline in nature while bitterness and the lesser vibrating emotions are acidic and can overstimulate stomach secretions. If someone is happy, brain and immune cells secrete hormones that resonate with happiness like endogenous opiates that go around boosting the immunity in the body wherever it is needed. The subtle energies of our emotions change the vibration of our overall physiology. Emotions trigger the simultaneous secretion of hormones all over the body. When we feel warm and loved, the veins and arteries are able to relax, dilate, and move blood, which increases circulation. When we feel cold and hated, depressed, or find ourselves in a state of fear, the blood slows down, breathing becomes shallow, and both the veins and arteries constrict. When this occurs it seems as though light has a more difficult time expressing itself through us.

Ch.39: Your Body Runs on Light

The human body as a living system which is structured in order to process light works the same way that the planet earth does in order to trap light in its many layers.

The human body makes use of apparently random light fluctuations. It is extremely intelligent and thermogenically regulates the temperature in us within a narrow margin that supports the body's maximum vitality levels. Our physical body is composed of electrons in perpetual motion. Life is composed of a blueprint that morphogenically causes the assemblage and manifestation of elements operating on the levels of neutrinos and electrons by way f biological transmutation.

Ions and conductive electrons each have unique radiation patterns. How fast or slow a person's pace and ease of moving is can generate an abundance of inner light or shut down this light quite dramatically. The more orderliness we have within the system the more intense the vacuum polarization effect is that harmonizes our whole body by strengthening the amplitude of the free flowing electrons. Either you have great amplitude of electricity to give you generous access to both sides of the brain and the frontal cortex or you operate from limited brain function that exhibits low amplitude of electricity with corresponding behaviors.

Diamagnetism is the interface of positive and negative polarities. Anionic elements are ions, predominately potassium, calcium, and chlorine that have spare electrons that spin centripetally to the left and are attracted toward the Van Alen belt in the sky. The minerals lithium, sodium, and calcium are biologically electropositive, while potassium sulfate, phosphate, and citrate are electronegative. The major electronegative center of the body is the thyroid gland. Due to its size, its amperage is small however its minerals give it a high voltage. Sodium can be deposited in the tissue of the thyroid and change its electromagnetic equilibrium, which is vital for homeostatic function. Electrons have a high affinity for oxygen, which is why they crowd at the surface, stimulating cellular respiration keeping the delicate balance of electrically negative cell membrane and its positive nucleus within.

Living cells radiate electrical potential into space surrounding them. With its perfect positive and negative magnetic composition, each cell has its own measurable electrical emission, vibrating from every place throughout the entirety of the body. Potassium is the intracellular colloidal ion and is electronegative in its surroundings, while sodium is biologically positive. Potassium likes to be near the positive nucleus while sodium prefers to be near the alkaline extracellular fluid. These +/- colloidal ions provide us with the ability to propagate electrical potential across the cell membrane. Colloidal minerals have been proven to activate enzyme systems throughout the body.

Each human cell is like a small wet battery. The principle of a wet cell battery is ionization and the release of hydrogen. Positive ions move towards the cathode (cations) in water solution while negative ions move towards the anode (anions). This principle works with organic cells of the mitochondria to store body electricity or universal life force energy. It appears in our body in the form of light and as its lesser degree in the form of electricity.

Electrons and protons act as if they love each other. Electrons appear to attract protons through their magnetic field. As any electrical charge moves it emits a magnetic field. As we said before, wherever there is light present, magnetism is there supporting it. Everything is caused as a result of light resonance and everything can also be thought of or understood as resonance itself. It is important to understanding that the more alive something is the more it is moving from the dense matter of nucleons and protons to the world of light and electrons. Having an abundant supply of electrons increase vitality. Both blood and lymph are referred to as isotonic fluids because the colloids they are composed of have spare electrons that keep basic forms of protein unobstructed and flowing.

Electrolytes are minerals in our body that carry an electric charge. Sodium, potassium, calcium, chloride, magnesium, and phosphorus are examples of electrolytes. They help us to maintain fluid balance since water always travels from a lower solute to a higher solute concentration. Coconuts are excellent sources and the electrolyte water in them is great for cleansing the bloodstream.

Ch.40: Your Blood Is Holographic

According to scientific experiments the average adult has approximately 9.55 pints of blood. In a healthy person, blood is the fourth heaviest organ after muscles, fat, and bone. It plays a huge role in nutrient delivery, waste management and life force distribution in our body. Blood is a liquid organ in and of itself when it is in its denser form but exists in more of a gas like state when the body is healthy and optimal. It streams through the vascular system, throughout the arteries, away from the heart to the arterioles to capillaries, and then returns via our veins to the heart once again. The lymphatic system involves managing the space between cells and clearing elements from between cells that would prevent them from otherwise fitting through our blood vessels. Together the blood and the lymph keep our body running like a constant cosmic event. Both of these fluid systems are of primary concern for those seeking to vitalize and improve the quality of the body.

Vitality is maintained as blood and lymph regulate the body like a wet cell battery. A blood cell is the most reactive in responding to our different states of consciousness. Blood serves as a connective tissue builder consisting of various types of cells in an extracellular fluid called plasma, which makes up about 50-60% of its volume. It carries gases, nutrients, hormones, and wastes around the body. Each platelet of blood is charged positively from the outer membrane and no two blood cells actually touch when the body is healthy as this positive charge has a repelling effect. The blood clots when this positive charge is lost due to foreign substances entering the body and consistent low levels of consciousness having a subtle but definite effect on the cells. About ninety percent of the body's plasma is made up of water with a plethora of different elements in it. The concentration of sodium, potassium, magnesium, and calcium determines the pH of the body fluids and tends to make the plasma slightly alkaline.

When the minerals iron and copper are out of balance our red blood cells loose their geometry and cellular integrity, which controls their ability to function and hold both water and nutrients. They also loose their ability to fit into the smaller capillaries in our body, which is what we see in people suffering from diabetes. Copper supplies our bodies with an electric charge while iron provides them with magnetism. They work in concert to create a foundation for the bulk of the human body's activities.

When the blood chemistry is altered it affects our entire being.

Formula for Blood Purification and Lymphatic System Revitalization
1 part Wakame
1 part Blue Flag
1 part Dandelion Root
1 part Kelp
1 part Dulse
1 part Horehound
1 part Cascara Sagrada
1 part Licorice
1 part Cat's Claw
2 parts Burdock root
1 part Prickly Ash
1 part Blood Root
1 part Red clover
1 part Camu Camu

In the same way the movie theatres use a machine to flash pictures on the screen rapidly to give the illusion of a motion picture, our more subtle nature projects itself out in the form of blood and ultimately the human body. This is a holographic universe and it is only our perception that makes us to believe that we are solid beings.

The Human Body

The human body is just a smaller, holographic reflection of Mother Nature and just as the Earth is mostly water making up the oceans, rivers, lakes and springs, we have our lymphatic system and bloodstreams to hydrate and nourish our own inner ecosystem. The earth breaths in air and vitality into its plants, animals, and landscapes, while we do the same with our lungs and veins as they deliver oxygen and life force energy to our own inner universe composed of cells, tissues and organs.

According to National Geographic, "Each cell in the human body contains about 100 times as many atoms as there are stars in the Milky Way."

The human body is a closed space with several openings. It has a definite mass, height, weight, depth, width, etc. unless altered via diet/substances, temperature, environment, patterns, lifestyle, innermost attitudes, or some effective external means. This allows for us to alter it at any given point in life making it of upmost importance for us to constantly remain self aware so that we are mindful of our condition at all times. Balance is the ideal condition for us to maintain and is the main prerequisite to achieving and preserving a healthy state of being. Even though we are responsible for the body that our spirit and mind occupies however we must also take into account the way other sentient beings are able to effect and influence us. Our body can be compartmentalized into various systems as shown in the charts throughout this book but it is ultimately composed in order to function as a single unit or form.

Everything going on it in whether on a small or large scale has an impact on everything else. This includes apparently obvious effects like harmful blows to the body or the consuming of meals and also seemingly insignificant phenomena like breathing or hearing music.

In chemistry, organic matter is generally defined as a carbon based material that exhibits systematic coordination of its molecular parts. Carbon is the primary building block of all living things on earth. It is a complex element that has the ability to bond with most elements. There a multiple groupings of carbon based molecules. Hydrocarbons are made from combinations of hydrogen and carbon. Amino compounds are made from combinations of carbon and nitrogen. Organometallics are made from combinations of carbon and metals. Organosilicons are made from combinations of carbon and silica. Most of these carbon-based molecules are able to bond with one another in systematic and coordinated patterns. These are the molecules that tend to make up the living tissue of plants and animals. These molecules are considered crystalline due to their ability to organize on a molecular level. This crystal attribute allows for them to have energy potential and to conduct, semi-conduct, and resonate with various energies just like other crystal materials. The crystalized molecules in a living body conduct the spirit or life force energy of the animating being inside them. The human body is composed of a variety of energy systems. These energy systems are composed of various crystal structures. These crystal structures are composed of molecules and so on and so on until we reach the most primordial levels of conscious within the person.

A system is defined as an organized group that works together as a functional unit. What we know of as the human body is actually highly organized and is made up of crystal structures working harmoniously as a wholesome machine. This complex crystal structure is made up of its composite organs, glands, tissues, bones, muscles, etc. These organic structures work together to maintain a balance of life force energy distributed throughout the entirety of the human body. The molecules making up our bodies are living and arranged in an energy network that enables us to conduct the universal life force energy. These crystalized molecules making up our bodies are carbon-based molecules that bond together in an organized pattern throughout our bodily systems. These molecules form a latticework or energy network that facilitates reception and transmission of life force energy throughout our structures and the body in its entirety.

There are three basic types of crystalized molecules and they are as follows from the simplest to the most complex. Mineral salts are ionic crystalized minerals often referred to as vitamins (living minerals). Biopolymers are chains of carbon-based molecules that have been bonded together. Hydrocarbons and amino compounds are the primary biopolymers in the human body. Melanin is an excellent example of a biopolymer. Deoxyribonucleic acid or DNA is a highly complex biopolymer composed of chains of less complex biopolymers. It is a giant crystalized molecule that is distinct from other biopolymers due to it containing encoded genetic information. This genetic information is inherited from ancestors via our parents and is the blueprint design for building the entire crystalized energy system that we call a human body.

Inside the human body, these diverse bio-crystalized molecules are arranged in the form of various mineral based structures. The primary crystalized structure in our body is a cell. Each cell contains all three bio-crystallized molecules: mineral salts, biopolymers, and DNA. The DNA in each cell is the blueprint for the cell's design. Depending on the genetic instructions, cells differentiate or change from one another to perform specific tasks in the body. Cells then group together to form more complex crystalized structured like blood, tissues, organs, skin, muscles and bones. The human body is a multilevel, multidimensional energy system and should be treated as such when striving to achieve greater states of health as opposed to simply targeting body parts or addressing symptoms.

Ions are the life carrier in our air supply and are necessary in our growth process to build cells. The human body cannot reproduce or regenerate a single cell without a supply of negative ions (available dielectricity). Ions are the first material manifestation of sunlight. The magnetic field of the Earth causes the X-ray and ultra-violet light from the sun to ionize. These hydrogen ions bind with one another as the building block of all other atomic structures. Hydrogen ions are the purest and finest form of the universal life force that we are aware of. Below the ionosphere, ions circulate abundantly as charged subatomic particles. They are considered "free" electrons that are not attached to atomic structures. These free ions are abundant around moving waters like bubbling streams, ocean beaches, waterfalls, and rivers. They exist in lesser amounts in large cities, urban areas, and places with higher levels of pollution in the air.

Many of the people occupying the world's hoods and our black and brown communities find themselves in environments that lack free ions. Toxicity is easy to find in these types of settings as the energy is found to be vibrating lower in these areas. A combination of pollution and ELFs devitalize the free ions available in the air. It is also a known fact that stressful urban lifestyles reduce ionic activities inside of our bodies. We should make it a point to adopt healthier practices to ensure that we maintain a condition with more free ions as opposed to toxins and free radicals.

Ions are essential to human vitality. The level of vitality and awareness a human has is directly related to the hydrogen ion levels of the blood plasma. High levels of hydrogen ions in the blood result in high levels of vitality and self-awareness. Low levels of hydrogen ions in our blood result in low levels of vitality and limited awareness. The more hydrogen ions a person has, the more potential they have to function, to regenerate, and to experience the highest of our emotional states.

The body's cell membranes are predominately composed these of hydrogen ions, which tend to be positively charged. This makes it so that negatively charged nutrients create maximum absorption the cell membranes. This is the process that the nutrients in our foods go through in the laboratories of our stomach and intestines in order to get into our blood. Nutrients are bound by protein carriers to become miscible with body fluids. The mineral components of these nutrients cross the cell membrane in a chelated form. Electrons flow from a positive pole toward a negative pole. The counterclockwise centripetal forces of an alkaline body create a state of implosion via a friction grid in which cosmic energy is condensed into electrons right inside of our bodies.

The body's biogenic field is beyond any ordinary field. Small portions of this energy have tremendous powers. The body's biogenic field is over 100 million times as large as its magnetic field. This biofield of energy produces force at right angles to the body. It appears in the form of spirals, without pushing or pulling like gravity or magnetic fields. The energy has the potential just like a scalper wave to reorganize the spin of electron clouds. This biofield of negative entropy creates order even out of systems that may seem to be inorganic.

Morphogenesis is the development of form and structure of the body and its parts. The same phenomenon occurs in plants and animals, as this field event is a means for the materialization that naturally occurs in all organisms in our universe. Morphogenesis comes from the Greek word "morphe" meaning shape and genesis meaning creation or generation. The term refers to the generation of form and is the biological process that causes a cell, tissue, or organism to develop its shape.

Biological transmutation is the ability to transmute one element into another alchemically i.e. organic silica into calcium, potassium into sodium, or manganese into iron.

Your Work

Ch.41: Authentic Body Building & Maintenance

When bodybuilding comes up, we typically think of people lifting weights or the increased consumption of protein and supplements. We also wrap our minds around some type of muscular system enhancement or alteration via various forms of external resistance. This is actually the effect of mass marketing with agendas including but not limited to selling massive amounts of proteins and the promotion of various sports. Real bodybuilding actually begins from within and continues throughout the durations of a lifetime. Although our genes play a huge role in the development of our physical bodies, the consciousness of a person assumes responsibility while the body is being developed and continues to intimately impact the body even after a person is finished growing. Our consciousness permeates and influences our subconscious mind, which in turn influences the subatomic particles in and around us. These subatomic particles obedient to our sub-consciousness, arrange themselves and manifest as atoms and as mentioned before these atoms go on to form molecules, cells, tissues, muscles, bodily systems, and ultimately an entire physical body. By remembering this sequential order when striving to improve our state of health, we can be more accurate and strategic with our methods resulting in a more definite or speedy recovery. If we continue to ignore this order then we are bound to repeat past mistakes and usher in new ones that are inevitable when we negate the very cause of all health and disease. With ego as the main culprit it is our very consciousness that's causes us to suffer either immediately or eventually in the long run.

Actual Order
Consciousness
Sub-consciousness
Subatomic particles
Atoms
Molecules
Cells
Tissues
Organs and Glands
Bodily Systems
Human Body
You

The real work done during a transformation is performed internally. Our minds are accustomed to dealing with the physical world at the level of effects versus placing our attention back at the level of causes. It should be understood at this point that the majority of modern day doctors and pharmaceutical companies address the body primarily with methods that are foreign to our body's natural rhythms.

Ch.42: Begin Where You Are

Thought is only the arrangement of the already present primordial material. When the body is polluted or not in shape (not in its ideal or sacred geometry) the said person will experience various levels of limitations and/or lack of comfort.

Move at your own realistic pace when manifesting a change in your state of health. Even though thoughts are instantaneous and are not restricted by the limits of time, evidence of the changes you make may manifest in intervals. Respect the law of graduality and watch as you progress on a daily basis. Trust yourself and trust the process. The truth is light and serves as an excellent purification method, mentally, as it allows the experiencer to discharge and let go of any false information. By being present with ones actual situation we can adjust and change things accordingly. Keep in mind that there is no such thing as the best diet for everyone. Each man or woman must walk his or her own path. We all need different types of fuel to fulfill our purpose. For example we may find individuals working together in a village but some may serve as warriors and guards while others are serving as midwives or doctors. These roles require different foods and personal practices for their respective outcomes. We highly recommend you seek out an understanding of the ancient art of *reduction.* There is no need to rush. Time is the measurement of magnitude and the movement of the celestial spheres i.e. planets. Be genuine and intentional and watch as you amaze those around you or even yourself.

A major mistake we make when striving to achieve health is limiting our attention to the level of effects as opposed to addressing the problem at its root. Medication for example stops the symptoms that patients have but the reason they felt the pain or discomfort in the first place is overlooked and eventually they will find themselves in a worse condition even after the doctor's "help". Many people confuse foods as the leading cause of disease or physical problems. While it is understandable as to why someone would come to this conclusion, it is still erroneous. The cause of our physical diseases is found in our consciousness. This is where we find the place that the food choices are made from. Consciousness is the distinguishing factor between a person who simple wants to eat for pleasure and a person who is choosing his or her foods to provide the body with what it needs.

Root Causes of Sickness and Death
Dehydration (Intensifies All Disease Phenomena)
Unhealthy Mitochondria (Reduces Vitality and Overall Functionality)
Colon Problems (Inhibits Circulation and Lowers Energy Levels)
Mucus Buildup (Creates a Breeding Ground for Toxins)
A Lack of Integrity (Disrespect of Maat Weakens the Body's Conductivity)
Fear (Cells Contract and Dismantle)
Worry (Magnetizes and Fuels Undesired Circumstances)
Stress (Weakens the Immune System)
Detrimental Environments (Cells Respond and Conform to Their Surroundings)
Poor Habits (Drain the Universal Life Force Energy)
Too Much Acidity (More Mass Than Spirit)

All true healers know and understand that diseases and problems of any sort must be addressed at the root. If the cause is not attended to then one can only expect temporary results if any are shown at all.

On Plants in General

Planets are endowed with immense magnetic powers and each of them acts upon the others in various ways according to their aspects and proximities. The sun is responsible for photosynthesis and life as we know it in the plant kingdom however, its influence is also accompanied by the rest of the planetary bodies in our solar system. The influences of the sun and planets vary on plants according to their chemical and elemental make-up. For example, plants containing high concentrations of iron are heavily influenced by the planet Mars while plants having a great concentration of zinc are predominantly influenced by Uranus. Plants are also multifaceted as they serve us in a wide variety of ways depending on the part we choose to consume and the environment that they were grown in. We group the vegetables according to the portion of the plant that they are derived from i.e. purple carrots (roots), lettuce (leaves), celery (stem), red onions (bulbs), etc. Fruits on the other hand are the most profound expression of the plants and their distinguishing factor is in their responsibility of carrying the seed. These are by far the most popular parts of the plant kingdom but the truth is that scientist and botanists haven't even discovered 10% of what the earth has to offer us. This means that we can eat a new fruit or vegetable for the rest of our lives and never run out of options. This also means that when it comes to gardening at home or farming in our communities that we have an abundance of options to choose from to insure our survival and our ability to sustain ourselves with Mother Nature's blessing.

Planetary and stellar forces magnetically endow all plants. The mineral composition and function of a plant are determined by the cosmic forces with the greatest influence on it. Some plants have multiple influences like peppermint, which is co-ruled by both Mars and Mercury. The word planet comes from the Greek word "planetes" meaning wanderer. The word plant comes from the Latin word "planta" meaning sprout or cutting and also from the French word "plantare" meaning to fix in a place.

Plants Rued By The Sun	Health Benefits
Acacia	Wound healing and restricting blood loss
Angelica	Overall circulatory system improvement
Bay Leaves	Antibacterial properties inhibition of E. coli
Bromeliad	Excellent source of fresh oxygen and clean air
Carnation	Stress relief and nervous system soothing
Cashew Fruit	Provider of nutrients for brain and bone health
Cedar	Antifungal, antiseptic and anti-inflammatory properties
Celandine	Eye health and throat cleansing
Centaury	Liver detoxer and blood purifier
Chamomile	Sleep, relaxation, and menstrual pain reduction
Chicory	Liver protection, stomach issues and constipation
Cinnamon	Antiviral, antibacterial, and antifungal properties
Citron	Excellent source of vitamin C and potassium
Eyebright	Eye health, headache relief and treatment for allergies
Frankincense	Combats asthma, oral health and arthritis
Goldenseal	Treatment for skin disorders and immunity issues
Hazel	Source of antioxidants and omega 3s
Heliotrope	Treatment for wounds and skin disorders
Lime	Edible electricity and ATP fuel
Marigold	Supports skin healing and reduces eye infections
Olive	Excellent source of vitamin e and healthy fats
Pineapple	Digestive enzymes and disease fighting antioxidants
Rosemary	Cognitive stimulant and memory enhancement
Saffron	Cancer fighting properties
Witch Hazel	Reduces skin irritation and inflammation

Plants Ruled By The Moon	Health Benefits
Adder's Tongue	Skin ulcer treatment and wound healing
Aloe	Improves skin and helps with wrinkles
Bladderwrack	Obesity, joint pain, constipation, and urinary tract
Cabbage	Lowers blood pressure and cholesterol levels
Camphor	Heals burns and treats arthritis
Chickweed	Treatment for wounds and skin ulcers
Coconut	MCTs, blood restoration and heart health
Cucumber	Promotes weight loss and hydration
Dulse	Bone, blood , eye and thyroid health
Eucalyptus	Cold symptoms and relaxation
Grapes	Vitamin C, vitamin K, and antioxidant properties
Jasmine	Improves oral health and brain function
Lemon	Edible electricity and ATP fuel
Lemon Balm	Boost cognition and relieves stress and anxiety
Lettuce	Excellent for hydration and vitamin A
Lotus Mallow	Urinary, digestive and respiratory health
Moonwort	Treatment for multiple sclerosis
Myrrh	Indigestion, colds, asthma, lung issues, and spasms
Papaya	Digestion, skin issues, and inflammation
Poppy	Headaches, coughs, and problems with asthma
Purslane	Beta-carotene, vitamin C, and omega 3s
Sandalwood	Bronchitis, diarrhea, fevers, and insomnia
Turnip	Vitamin B6, calcium, copper, and potassium
Willow	Gout, headaches, muscle pain, and joint pain
Wintergreen	Rheumatism, sore muscles, and lower back pain

Plants Ruled By Mercury	Health Benefits
Almond	Vitamin E, magnesium, and healthy fats
Aspen	Rheumatoid arthritis and nerve pain
Beans	Diabetes and glucose metabolism
Bittersweet	Eczema, itchy skin, acne, boils, and warts
Bracken	Insomnia and fever treatment
Brazil Nut	Selenium, antioxidants, and inflammation reduction
Caraway	Heartburn, digestive problems, bloating & gas issues
Celery	Digestion, inflammation and body alkalization
Clover	Respiratory issues, coughs, and skin disorders
Dill	Vitamin C, vitamin A, and magnesium
Fennel	Vitamin B6, potassium, and phytonutrients
Fenugreek	Blood sugar levels and milk production
Fern	Sore throat, colds, measles, and tuberculosis
Lavender	Promotes calmness and wellness
Lemongrass	Bacteria and yeast growth prevention
Mace	Diarrhea, nausea, stomach spasms, and pain
Mandrake	Stomach ulcers, constipation, asthma, & hay fever
Mulberry	Excellent source of iron and vitamin C
Papyrus	Eye diseases and ulcers
Parsley	Kidney, heart, and bone health
Pecan	Brain health and blood pressure issues
Pistachio	Fiber and unsaturated fats
Pomegranate	Antioxidants and cancer prevention
Senna	Digestive problems and weight loss
Wax Plant	Pollution remover in an indoor environment

Plants Ruled By Venus	Health Benefits
Adam and Eve	Anemia, joint pain, tumor prevention, diarrhea
African Violet	Increases oxygen to brain, energy booster, relaxation
Alder	Sore throat, fevers, swelling, and excess bleeding
Alfalfa	Copper, folate, magnesium, vitamin C, vitamin K
Apple	Fiber, digestive health, diabetes, heart health
Apricot	Eye and skin health, liver and gut health, potassium
Avocado	Vitamin, C, vitamin E, vitamin B6, vitamin K, omega 3s
Balm of Gilead	Anti-inflammatory, antifungal, helps to reverse cancer
Burro Banana	Digestion, weight loss, and antioxidants
Birch	Kidney & bladder health, vitamin C, urinary infections
Blackberry	Oral health, brain health, vitamin C, vitamin K
Bleeding Heart	Increases appetite, stimulates liver metabolism
Blue Flag	Bloating, fluid retention, swelling, skin problems
Burdock	Removes toxins from blood, antioxidant property
Caper	Manganese, calcium, niacin, vitamin E, vitamin A
Cardamom	Antioxidant, antibacterial, cancer fighting components
Catnip	Relaxation, anxiety, nervousness, and depression
Cherry	Improves quality of sleep, arthritis, inflammation
Coltsfoot	Gout, respiratory issues, brain damage, and fevers
Cowslip	Swollen nose and throat, colds, coughs, hysteria
Daffodil	n/a (toxic to humans)
Daisy	Coughs, bronchitis, liver disorders, kidney issues
Elder	Stress reduction, heart health, immunity, flu symptoms
Feverfew	Uterine contractions, inflammation, arthritis
Foxglove	Congestive heart failure, headaches, constipation

Plants Ruled By Mars	Health Benefits
Allspice	Indigestion, intestinal gas, vomiting, and diarrhea
Basil	Improved cognition, memory enhancement, anxiety
Black Snakeroot	(In small amounts) vaginal dryness, vertigo, hot flashes
Blood Root	Tooth pain, circulation, warts, fevers, and colds
Cactus	Stroke, coronary heart disease, and blood pressure
Chili Pepper	Improves circulation, digestion and metabolism
Coriander	Antioxidants, brain and heart health, digestion
Cumin	Antibacterial, anti-parasitic, anti-inflammatory
Curry Leaf	Weight loss, diabetes, eyesight, stress reduction
Damiana	Aphrodisiac, treatment for headaches, depression
Dragon's Blood	Antibacterial, antifungal, and antiviral
Garlic	Blood thinner when used in moderation
Ginger	Curbs cancer growth, nausea, digestive health
Hawthorn	Heart health, circulation, blood pressure, skin problems
Hops	Anxiety, ADHD, insomnia, and sleeping disorders
Horseradish	Helps to prevent lung, stomach, and colon cancers
Masterwort	Stomach disorders, swelling, digestive problems
Mustard	Phosphorus, zinc, iron, manganese, and calcium
Nettle	Enlarged prostate issues, hay fever, blood sugar
Onion	Nervous system restoration and inflammation
Peppermint	Energy boost, digestive health and bacterial infections
Pine	Inflammation, stuffy nose, blood pressure problems
Prickly Ash	Toothaches, sores, ulcers, and joint pain
Shallot	Antioxidants, circulation, and bone health
Thistle	Brain function and liver protection

Plants Ruled By Jupiter	Health Benefits
Agrimony	Cancers, gall bladder disorders, and IBS
Anise	Anti fungal, antibacterial, and anti-inflammatory
Avens	Diarrhea, colitis, uterine bleeding, and fevers
Banyan	Antioxidant support and blood sugar levels
Bodhi	Snake bites, asthma, and kidney diseases
Borage	Increased urine flow, inflammation and depression
Chestnut	Cardiovascular issues, magnesium, and potassium
Cinquefoil	PMS, soreness, and swelling
Clove	Free radical fighter and parasite killer
Dandelion	Blood purifier and liver cleanser
Dock	STDs and intestinal infections
Endive	Weight loss, blood regulation, and pregnancy
Figs	Copper, magnesium, potassium, and vitamin K
Honeysickle	Urinary disorders, headaches, diabetes, and arthritis
Horse Chestnut	Varicose veins and enlarged prostate treatment
Houseleek	Severe diarrhea, burns, ulcers, and warts
Hyssop	Intestinal pain, coughs, and respiratory infections
Linden	Nasal congestion, fevers, and colds
Liverwort	Blood circulation and purification
Maple	Brain health and manganese deficiency prevention
Meadowsweet	Upset stomach, heartburn, peptic ulcer disease
Nutmeg	Excellent for cognitive function if used in small doses
Sage	Antioxidants, oral health, and blood sugar levels
Sarsaparilla	Joint pain, inflammation and skin irritation
Witch Grass	Repels positive ions in surrounding areas

Plants Ruled By Saturn	Health Benefits
Amaranth	Calcium, magnesium, and copper
Asphodel	Cough remedy and skin healing
Beets	Prostate health, blood flow and manganese
Belladonna	Parkinson's disease and inflammatory bowel disease
Bistort	Digestive problems and throat infections
Buckthorn	Vitamin C, heart health, and liver support
Comfrey	Sprains, strains, pulled muscles, and inflammation
Cypress	Hemorrhoids and varicose veins
Datura	Fevers, heart health, and fertility
Euphorbia	Asthma, bronchitis, and chest congestion
Hellebore	Treatment for gout and high blood pressure
Hemlock	Breathing problems and pain relief
Hemp	Heart health, omega 3s and omega 6s
Hembane	Muscle tremors and digestive problems
Kava-Kava	Pain relief and seizure prevention
Knot Weed	Bronchitis, cough, and gingivitis
Lady's Slipper	Insomnia, anxiety, nervousness and hysteria
Lobelia	Asthma, bronchitis, pneumonia
Mimosa	Antibacterial, anti-venom, and antidepressant help
Morning glory	Laxative, diuretic, and blood purifier
Mullein	Tuberculosis, bronchitis, allergies, and sore throats
Skunk Cabbage	Ringworms, fluid retention, snakebites, and skin sores
Slippery Elm	Inflammatory bowel conditions
Tamarind	Pineal gland cleansing and gut health

Entheogen

(Oxford Dictionary)

From Greek, literally 'becoming divine within'.

As we study the health, nutrition, and nature in general it become quite obvious that specific plants work to heal and address specific parts of the body. We see that plants like dandelion root, burdock root, and milk thistle all help to heal different aspects of the liver. Likewise, plants such as hawthorne berry, cacao beans, olives, coconuts, and avocados all help to heal and restore aspects of the heart and our cardiovascular system. There is no category of food in existence that is more powerful when it comes to healing and strengthening our minds than entheogens also known as the power plant family. They have the unique ability to penetrate the blood brain barrier and introduce potent medicinal alkaloid compounds as well as rare phytochemicals, which stimulate the regeneration, synchronization and detoxification of our brain cells and corresponding hemispheres. Simultaneously these amazing plants also work to stimulate our pineal gland, which is responsible for producing the world famous hormones, serotonin and melatonin. Entheogens are highly recommended no matter what type a diet you may choose for yourself.

Section 9 Summary

Whether we are talking about physical exercise, mental exercise, or spiritual exercise, I lean towards a saying I've heard at the dojo during training – *"Master movement, master life."* In the above section, Asa is speaking on movement. When there's no movement, there is a block which will clog you up and cause problems.

The healthiest people are all focusing on constant movement which despite popular belief, starts from the top (the spirit) on down (the body). Being in tune with yourself means you can move consciousness (spirit) properly, influencing movement of your limbs. Having a strong vessel (body) allows you to move consciousness effectively. Your mind is the key to unlock your physical abilities. Having a sharp mind means you will have a sharp body. It's a circular dynamic when it comes to the work needed – exercise the spirit, mind, then body.

Starting where you are is important in this section. More important, start your journey for you, not in the resemblance of someone else's journey. Often, we tend to start our journey where we've seen others start theirs. "I want to look like Dewayne "The Rock" Johnson," when I should want to look like myself. In wanting to look like

The Rock, many will start their journey according to what The Rock said he started his journey. Knowing who you are will equip you to know where you are. Knowing where you are will equip you with the ability to take steps towards optimal that fits YOU. Everyone has a different path towards optimal health because we are all positioned differently. Although the process is the same, we are all in a different mental and spiritual space. So, you must understand where you are to start your journey.

Special Foods

Ch.43: On Sea Vegetables

Seaweed and *Algae* can be found all over the world and are excellent sources of nutrition for not only aquatic animals but humans as well. Seaweed is the umbrella term for the entire group of macro algae living in salt water, brackish water, or fresh water. Algae is the term for some of the macro algae but it is typically used to refer to the micro algae (unicellular organisms like chlorella). They have survived under the most severe circumstances known to man and serve as a source of food and indirect sustenance for sentient beings on earth. They too practice photosynthesis and are responsible for the majority of oxygen (85%)on our planet enabling life to exist, as we know it. There are tens of thousands of species of algae that have been named and classified so far while new species are still being discovered to this day. We can find seaweed in every large body of water whether it's warmer by the equator or ice cold by the poles.

Green Algae derives its name from its color and lives in both salt water and freshwater. These algae prefer nutrient rich waters with high concentrations of phosphate and nitrate. Green algae contain the same photogenic pigments as land plants, chlorophyll a and chlorophyll b. One of the most commonly found forms of green algae is the *Ulva*, or sea lettuce, which can be found near the east and west coasts of the Americas, among other bodies of water.

Brown Algae are almost exclusively salt water species and can rarely be found in fresh water. Most of the brown algae live in the cold waters of the Northern Hemisphere. One of the largest algae of any type is a brown algae known as *Kelp*, which can grow up to 200 feet long and is found near southern Alaska. Worldwide there are estimated to be over 2,000 species of brown algae.

Red Algae vary in color from pink to dark red and sometimes even purple or reddish black. The color is determined by the amount of red pigment in the seaweed. These algae do contain the green pigment, chlorophyll but they are dominated by the red pigments, phycocyanin and phycoerythrin. About 6,500 species of red algae are known to man and these are the best suited for the deeper waters as they absorb the blue light from the sunlight spectrum. They tend to live and thrive in warmer waters and can be found in abundance in Asia. Red algae are most used for consumption due to their nutritional value and availability. The seaweed in sushi, nori, is a red algae.

At one point in time, seaweed was considered a luxury product due to its healing properties. In our modern world it is still an important part of Ayurvedic medicine in India and other parts of the planet that practice the craft. Algae have been used as medication in China and japan for thousands of years and seaweed was and still is a substantial part of the everyday diet there and many other countries that practice traditional herbal medicine. Seaweed is regarded as a treatment for tuberculosis, rheumatism, colds, open wounds, and even intestinal worms. It is even ranked as one of the world's so called *super foods*.

Kelp or *Kombu*, again, is the most well known brown algae and is sometimes referred to as the "King of the sea." It is used a lot of many Japanese, Chinese, and Korean dishes and can be eaten in several forms i.e. dried, fresh, roasted, frozen, cooked, stir-fried, marinated or candied. Like most seaweed, the taste and texture of the kelp varies depending on the species and the age. It is also an excellent salt substitute for individuals and societies who tend to consume more sodium than necessary.

Wakame is brown algae native to Asian waters and ranges in color from olive green to brown. The individual leaves are long, rubbery, and smooth while the taste is described as soft and sweet. Wakame has less iodine than other brown algae but is an excellent source of calcium. Raw and marinated Wakame is matched well with vegetable salads and stir-fries.

Hijiki or *Hiziki* is another brown algae and is native to the Pacific coats of Japan. It is harvested in the spring and has small leaves resembling tea. Be sure to research and find hijiki from uncontaminated waters as they are known to store elevated levels of arsenic, which in high concentrations is poisonous to humans.

Arame is a brown algae that grows on both sides of the Pacific Ocean as well as in South America. It lives on open rocky coasts and prefers cold waters. In order to dry Arame it is laid out and cooked in the sun then sliced in to strips. It is very dark and sometimes can even come across as black but turns brown after it is submerged in water and like some other algae, it significantly increase in volume. Arame contains plenty of calcium, iron, magnesium, and vitamins A abd B3. It has a very subtle taste and can be used in a variety of dishes ranging from salads to soups to stews.

Sea Spaghetti or "Thongweed" is also a brown algae and grows mainly on the Irish, British, and French coasts as well as the Baltic Sea. This algae is known for its elongated greenish brown cords which can be many feet in length depending on its age and the quality of the water it's found in. They are found to be the tastiest when they are harvested in the spring. The sea spaghetti can be enjoyed raw and has a salty but smooth flavor. This algae is rich in dietary fibers, vitamins A,C and E and also iron. It serves as an excellent substitute for pasta dishes.

Dulse is a red algae that grows predominantly on the northern coasts of the Pacific and Atlantic oceans. It can also be found near Russia, Canada, and Alaska as well as many Asian coasts. Dulse fluctuates between red, brown, and purple but can also embody a combination of these colors. The texture of its leaves resemble leather and like the majority of algae, it is best when harvested at the end of the summer. In order to be made more bioavailable for consumption, it must first be rinsed and then dried out in the sun, which eventually brings its salt content to the surface. It has both a soft and a crunchy bite and contains more protein then most poultry and nuts.

Nori or *Purple Seaweed* is the most popular and most frequently used seaweed in the world today. Nori is harvest from the beginning of spring up until the summer. The familiar green color is only found after the nori has been roasted. It is most commonly used for sushi rolls, but it is also delicious when bean combinations, vegetables, pastas, and wild rice. It has high protein content and contains large amounts of iodine, carotene, and also vitamins A,B, and C.

Irish Moss or *Chondrus Crispus* is a red algae that grows about 8 inches and is known to be a source to be a source of carrageenan although there are about 40 different varieties all of which do not contain this carbohydrate. Chondrus crispus has been shown to hold up to 200 times its weight in water and can be used as a stabilizer and thickener in both drinks and food dishes.

Sea Lettuce is a green algae native to the coastal zones of all the world's oceans. It lives and thrives in nutrient rich environments and can grow all year round but is most abundant in the summer. The leaves are think, firm, and irregular in shape. Sea lettuce is an annual plant and dies off around the autumn season. This is typically the time when it is found in bulk on the shorelines. For hundreds of years, this seaweed has been used as a natural fertilizer. It contains magnesium, calcium, vitamin A, and vitamin C. It is relatively high in protein and low in fat making it ideal for salads and a variety of other meals.

Sea Vegetables get their distinctive and fascinating taste from the ocean and seawater. These plants grow on land and have a strong resistance to salt water. They actually live on the border between the land and the sea. Their greatest similarity to seaweed is that they contain many vitamins and minerals from the ocean and they are easily assimilated into our bodies making them an ideal source of key nutrients.

Samphire is a salt-tolerant, annual plant from the amaranth family. Like the cactus, samphire is a succulent, which is a type of plant known found to be more resistant to drought than other land plants. It is native to North America and the western portions of Asia, where it grows in salt marshes and on beaches. It is a small green plant, usually less than 8 inches, with a strong stem and straight branches. It is also called glasswort, pickleweed, and marsh samphire. It has a pronounced salty flavor and tastes similar to baby spinach.

Sea Aster is a plant belonging to the sunflower family. This species lives around the high-tide lines and thrives on soils with a relatively high salt content. It can found in north Africa, Russia, and China and changes colors from green to red in autumn. The shape of its leaves is where its nickname, lamb's ear, is derived. Te leaves are typically eaten while the plant is still young as this stage has proven to be the most bioavailable to humans.

Oyster Leaf, which is also called sea blueshells or oyster plant, grows along the beaches of North Africa and the East Asia. It is native to salty environments and changes in color from red to light blue. By the time it reaches full bloom, it looks more like an herb than a sea vegetable. It has a crunchy bite and the taste resembles that of an oyster, thus its name. Steaming this plant is best to retain its taste and texture and the roots can be consumed as well after they have been cooked.

Sea Kale is related to the cabbage family and is native to East Asia. This plant perseveres and thrives in places where other plants wouldn't survive. It can be found in freezing temperatures and salty soils. It is fragile and difficult to transport but is worth the challenge as it offers a salty-nutty taste. It can be consumed fresh upon harvesting with an exception of its green leafy portion.

Sea Fennel can be found in the Black Sea, the Mediterranean Sea, the Canary Islands, and the Atlantic Ocean. It can grow anywhere from 8 to 20 inches and has a woody stem with short, thick leaves. Sea fennel is sold by specialized growers and contains essential oils, which give it a unique flavor. Only its fleshly leaves are edible and it is typically consumed in salads and other vegetable based dishes.

Sea Beet is a member of the amaranth family is the wild ancestor of modern vegetables like sugar beets, regular beets, and Swiss chard. This plant grows primarily in East Asia and Northern Africa but can also be found on the Mediterranean coast. The sea beet requires moist, moderately salty soil, and grown anywhere between 12 and 32 inches. It has a salty and nutty flavor and only its leaves are edible. The younger leaves are more pleasant while the adult leaves are bitter. When preparing in dishes it has shown to be the most pleasant when steamed.

(Phytoplankton, algae, and plants deliver minerals to us in the most assimilative form.)

*There are elements in blue-green algae macrophage activity that helps diseased bodies go into remission and shrink tumors. Interferon production is stimulated in the body, providing phytochemicals that help repair DNA.

Blue-green algae also contain significant GACs (carbohydrates linked to a core protein). There are even steroid like compounds found abundantly in living foods like algae that help to moderate cholesterol and lower viscous blood fats while simultaneously strengthening the tissue of our body and keeping it anchored together in a healthy manner. EFAs are similar substances to our hormones that are produced locally by cells. Omega-3 essential fatty acids supply the precursors to make prostaglandins. These substances are involved with nearly every bodily function.

Forces in Foods

We understand that all diseases are the result of us being out of order with nature, which causes a lack of electrical vitality or energy potential at the cellular level. In other words there is an overall lack of nerve force. In order to combat this we can look to foods like uncooked fruits and vegetables, soaked and sprouted nuts and seeds, or direct sunlight. Organic and in-season fresh produce are great options or they can be properly dried and stored for later use. It is ideal to consume foods than can reproduce themselves in nature. Most foods from Mother Nature are already prepared to be easily digestible. The enzymes present in naturally grown foods have a survival temperature of 118 degrees Fahrenheit and if they are cooked above and beyond this point, the enzymes will be reconfigured. Energy and nutrients will still be provided however one should not expect to receive the same level of benefit as would be the case if the food was left in its original state. It is important to understand that enzymes are necessary for digestion to occur. If food is without enzymes the body must scavenge from its personal supply to digest whatever nutrients there are in the foods eaten. When we borrow from important enzyme reserves within our body, it manifests as the process of aging. We witness the reversal of this aging process whenever we fast strictly on living foods for at least 72 hours. The standard American diet is not just in America now and typically consists of white sugars, excess starch, rancid oil, and processed denatured foods which have taken a toll on the health and vitality of our people all over the world.

The minerals in the food we eat and how close they are to biological transmutation into mold, fungus, and yeast is important to take into account when understanding what contributes to disease phenomena. Tar, resin, and glue-like acid forming substances from cooked milk, excess amounts of grain, pastas, breads, and too much cooked flesh can cause adhesions in the body and obstruction in blood vessels and lymphatic spaces. These food choices also cause build up in bile ducts and in and around the intestinal tract binding everything together, which obstructs the flow of our vital life forces. None of these foods mentioned should be thought of as "bad", however they should be eaten in moderation or balanced out every now and then with some form of bodily cleansing if one is interested in creating a healthy physical body.

Natural vital foods have a measurable force field, which can be identified and made visible by Kirlian photography. An apple fresh from a tree or bush for example can be witnessed radiating a living field of energy extending well beyond its skin but if we were to cook the apple or place it in a microwave we would notice that this same field becomes diminished or even unnoticeable. Consuming natural vital foods even for a short period of time provides one with experimental proof in itself how quickly the body heals when it is given the proper nourishment of the wholesome vitamins and minerals. The body is a perfect self-correcting machine. We are physical, mental, emotional, and spiritual beings and health is a matrix of these aspects that changes and fluctuates during the course of life according to the choices we make.

"Fruits provide the body with the greatest fuel and do the best job of cleansing the cells."

" Vegetables are excellent for providing the body with structure and cellular integrity."

"Herbs are excellent for healing and regenerating the body."

"Ancient grains are great for building mass and muscle tissues."

"What is a weed? A plant whose virtues have not yet been discovered."

–Ralph Waldo Emerson

Section 10 Summary

Asa will deep dive in general nutrition later. In regard to this section, Solonic Botanicals and Amazon are reputable places to find most of or all of the described special foods.

Mother Earth

Ch.44: Mother Nature

Mother Nature is like an energy sink. When a rock or a dense enough object falls into a lake or a pool of water and creates a void, the water produces waves in response. The energy in the wave travels outwards from the center in circle. The same amount of energy is in each ring but in the large more expanded rings, the energy is more dispersed throughout the entirety of the wave. The intensity is decreased as the rings increase in size. Our consciousness works the exact same way and works in accordance with this law. The further from the seat of consciousness, the weaker the energy becomes except in cases where the individual is capable of placing his or her thinking above and beyond both space and time in order to have a more instant effect on people, things, or circumstances. The one thing that is common is that Mother Nature is responsive and receptive to us and will react in direct correspondence to the ways that we interact with her whether it be spiritually, mentally, or physically.

When we step outside of the box that the western world has presented to us by spending more time in wild forests, mountains, beaches, and other natural places, we are allowed to re-experience the magic that Mother Nature has to offer and to tap back into the real world behind the illusions that we were taught to fuel with our modern-day habits and lifestyles. We stimulate our original state of mind when we begin to re-establish a relationship with her (Mother Nature). We reconnect to our deeper levels of sensory perception of that which is both in and around us. This type of natural sense of awareness and perception is often blunted and altered by the constant activities carried on around us in our modern urban settings. We can unlock this power however when we clean up our acts and do a better job of harmonizing with Mother Nature as she patiently waits for us to blend back into the natural order of the universe.

In the ancient ennead we find that our ancestors had developed a system whereby they could comprehend the nature of anything in existence. They used anthropomorphism to show the relationship between the basic elements, their qualities, and the relationships that they have with each other. Their art and teachings correspond with the nature of elements as we know them today and the ways they combine to produce change in the atmosphere. For example, like we previously stated, when we combine moisture with cold, we get water or when we combine cold with dry, we get earth and so on. Unity however is the principle underlying all things and is the most powerful force known to man. In some way form or fashion all things emanate from it, so the harmonization of these elements is where we see the most profound manifestations of nature.

Mother Nature has a tendency to form circles since she is an extension of such a wholesome creative force. Cells are an excellent example of this and are outstanding resonators, emitting, and absorbing radiation. Our blood emits and absorbs radiation of the highest frequency in the body. Disease manifests itself out of a desperate need for cell oscillatory stability and harmony inside. Maintaining vital cell vibration is the ley to reversing diseased states in us. Cell nuclei are electrical oscillating circuits and DNA filaments within the nuclei oscillate according to specific frequencies. Cells and larger life forms possess a sink that enables a direct tapping into cosmic radiation, which allows us to oscillate according to various ranges of vibration. All our cells vibrate with their own personal signature. In a healthy body they vibrate harmoniously like an orchestra. Resonating with the Earth greatly speeds up the healing process.

Excellent hygiene is one of Mother Nature's most fascinating features. Dominating one's diet with foods straight from her is a sure and simple means of creating order inside the body if the innermost attitude of the person is pristine enough. Nature is inherently wise so when we eat foods in their natural state this wisdom is transferred and delivered into our body. Our bodies being miniaturized versions of the universe have an affinity with nature and our immune systems can identify the codes embedded inside of the foods we eat if they are derived from Mother Nature. Processed and manufactured foods on the other hand give our bodies a hard time and are seen as outsiders resulting in various degrees of immune responses.

Universal principles can be observed in Mother Nature. Atmospheric electric activity gathers itself in points and spirals, orchestrating an ion exchange between the Earth and the sky. There are reservoirs deep within us that are in resonance with celestial energy from the furthest reaches of outer space. Massive fission reactors occurring in the celestial stars and our Sun provide our body with unlimited potential that can be tapped into.

"Science cannot solve the ultimate mystery of nature. And that is because, in the last analysis, we ourselves are a part of the mystery that we are trying to solve." –Max Planck

If we continue to seek answers outside of ourselves, we will find ourselves with results that are incomplete. If we would only look inward for solutions to our challenges and problems, we would see that the greatest remedies to issues we face come about when we acknowledge and honor our roles in the grand scheme of things. We are here for significant reasons and an examination of self must be made to the same degree that we study and analyze things outside of us. We must also keep in mind that there are levels to our inner world so there is no need to stop searching and discovering once a layer is identified and understood.

On George Washington Carver

George Washington Carver is most popular for the multitude of benefits he shared in regard to the peanut. George Washington Carver was an agricultural scientist and inventor who reminded us of how magical Mother Nature is. He was a botanist and conducted experiments in plant pathology (diseases of plants). He also dealt with the cultivation of superior soil for farming and gardening. He showed that it was possible to not only improve the quality of soil but to integrate crops and plant them in sequential orders to get the best use out of the nutrients left behind. His contribution makes it easy for us to become much more creative in our relationship with nature. He discovered over 100 products that could be developed from the sweet potato so just imagine what we can accomplish in today's world if we put our time and attention back into creation as opposed to allowing ourselves to being brainwashed by the digital world.

On Benjamin Banneker

Benjamin Bannecker's contributions to the modern world were unparalleled during his lifetime. Benjamin Banneker was born on a farm outside of Baltimore, Maryland in 1731. He was a polymath and shared his gifts with the world as an astronomer, mathematician, surveyor, and Master Mason. He is responsible for designing the city layout for Washington, D.C. and even advised presidents of the United States. In this book however we want to highlight his popularization of the almanac as it has shown to be pivotal in the field of agriculture. Benjamin Banneker has impacted the world in so many ways that we take for granted but his legacy will live on thru the works of those that he continues to inspire.

Almanacs serve as an excellent source of information to benefit not only gardeners and farmers but the normal person as well who may want to go about planting and tending to their homegrown foods in the best possible manner. Weather forecasts, planting dates, tide tables, moon cycles, and planetary positions are some of the most well-known features found in most almanacs. We recommend them when starting out at home and especially in community gardens so that the participants can be on one accord.

While following instructions from professionals are ideal, it is also important to pay attention to your crops throughout their development to respond to them in the best way possible. These are just few examples of what that looks like.

Problem	Reason	Solution
Long and pale leaves	Not enough light	More sunlight
Leaves curl underneath	Too much light	Less light or put them in some shade
Mushy stems	Too much water	Water only when soil is dry
Brown leaf tips	Not enough water	Soak pot for 20 minutes then drain
Leaf edges are crinkly	Lack of humidity	Mist the leaves
Lower leaves falling off	Lack of fertilizer	Use an all-natural fertilizer

Ch.45: On Soil

While most people try to avoid getting dirty, there are countless scientific studies that show that ingesting soil because of inhalation by accident can drastically improve brain functioning. Children's immune systems are also shown to be stronger in those who play around in dirt as opposed to those who are sheltered and spend most of their time in closed doors. What has also been discovered is that a specific strain of bacteria called, *Mycobacterium Vaccae*, stimulates brain cells to produce large amounts of the neurotransmitter serotonin, and can provide an antidepressant like effect. This type of soil bacteria is not harmful and can be referred to as "friendly bacteria." To add more of these beneficial bacteria to your life, take up gardening, go hiking in nature, or simple spend more time out in nature. Dirt is not only good for the brain but is also a key ingredient which allows oxygen producing trees and food bearing plants to live and thrive.

Most soil formation is the direct result of living organisms working to create the proper living conditions for themselves. Rots and small soil organisms use several chemical forces like oxidation, reduction, carbonation, etc. in order to modify the soil, while roots and different burrowing animals act as mechanical forces to mix and reassemble it. In just a teaspoon of soil we can find billions of microorganisms carrying on different life functions i.e., metabolism, respiration, reproduction, dying, excreting hormones and enzymes, exchanging cations and anions, responding to cosmic forces like lunar phases and sun cycles. Soil is not a single thing but is a combination of potencies and organisms that work together collectively to manifest the best possible display of cohesion.

Organism in the soil have the job of recycling nutrients, regulating pH levels, aerating the soil, chelating minerals, and eventually creating crumbly, good-smelling earth that can support the vegetation. They are also capable of decomposing certain forms of liter by reducing proteins and related substances to NH4 and NO3 that can be taken up by growing plants. Some of them produce sulphates, which are the most important for of Sulphur utilized by higher reaching plants. Some of the autotrophic organisms oxidize iron and magnesium, avoiding toxic build-ups in the soil, while others can fix atmospheric nitrogen.

Simple Ways To Test Your Soil
Laboratory Test
Self-Test
Earthworm Test
Pantry Test

Be sure to test your soil if you are unsure of its quality. Laboratory tests can be done if you live in a city, or you can even find a source online to ship the soil to. They typically cost around $20.00 plus shipping fees for the process. You can also use self-test kits that can be purchased for even less. These kits test the soils pH level as well as the nitrogen, phosphorus, and potassium content and usually come with some sort of color coding for you to differentiate between healthy and damaged soil. Earthworms are a good indicator of healthy soil as they tend to thrive in quality and search elsewhere or die off when the vibration of the soil is not up to par. If you find little to no earthworms, you may want to add some organic matter immediately followed by constant nourishing throughout the year as you between to recondition the area you are utilizing. You can test the pH of your soil right at home in your pantry as well. Put about 2 tablespoons of soil into a bowl or glass can ½ cup of vinegar. If the mixture fizzes up, then this indicates alkalinity in the soil. To test for acidity, you can use the same about of soil but moisten it slightly with distilled water then add about a ½ cup of baking soda. If it fizzes, then this is an indication of acidity in the soil. If you find that your soil doesn't react to either test, then you have soil with a neutral pH.

Most plants thrive in a pH range between slightly acidic and neutral. Some plants are more sensitive than others but as with all crops it can't be stressed enough how important it is to monitor your plants and t develop your own personal relationship with them. Applying finely ground limestone can counteract acidic soil and alkaline soil can be balanced by grounded sulfur. The following charts will serve to show how plants have their own requirements from the soil and the environment around them.

Trees and Shrubs	Ideal pH Range
Apple	5.0-6.5
Azalea	4.5-6.0
Beautybush	6.0-7.5
Birch	5.0-6.5
Blackberry	5.0-6.0
Blueberry	4.0-5.0
Boxwood	6.0-7.5
Sour Cherry	6.0-7.0
Crab Apple	6.0-7.5
Hemlock	5.0-6.0
Hydrangea (Blue-Flowered)	4.0-5.0
Hydrangea (Pink-Flowered)	6.0-7.0
Juniper	5.0-6.0
Laurel (Mountain)	4.5-6.0
Lemon	6.0-7.5
Lilac	6.0-7.5
Maple	6.0-7.5
Oak (White)	5.0-6.5
Orange	6.0-7.5
Peach	6.4-8.0
Plum	6.0-8.0

Flowers	Ideal pH Range
Alyssum	6.0-7.5
England	6.0-8.0
Baby's Breath	6.0-7.0
Bee Balm	6.0-7.5
Begonia	5.5-7.0
Bleeding Heart	6.0-7.5
Canna	6.0-8.0
Carnation	6.0-7.0
Chrysanthemum	6.0-7.5
Clematis	5.5-7.0
Coleus	6.0-7.0
Cosmos	5.0-8.0
Daffodil	6.0-6.5
Foxglove	6.0-7.5
Geranium	6.0-8.0
Hibiscus	6.0-8.0
Marigold	5.5-7.5
Peony	6.0-7.5
Snapdragon	5.5-7.0
Sunflower	6.0-7.5
Tulip	6.0-7.0

Fruits and Vegetables	Idea pH Range
Asparagus	6.0-8.0
Beet	6.0-7.5
Broccoli	6.0-7.0
Cabbage	6.0-7.5
Carrot	5.5-7.0
Celery	5.8-7.0
Chive	6.0-7.0
Eggplant	6.0-7.0
Leek	6.0-8.0
Lettuce	6.0-7.0
Okra	6.0-7.0
Onion	6.0-7.0
Potato	4.8-6.5
Pumpkin	5.5-7.5
Radish	6.0-7.0
Spinach	6.0-7.5
Squash (Crookneck)	6.0-7.5
Squash (Hubbard)	5.5-7.0
Swiss Chard	6.0-7.0
Tomato	5.5-7.5
Watermelon	5.5-6.5

Ch.46: The Secret Life Of Plants

In 1973, Peter Tompkins wrote a paradigm-shifting book using this title. "The Secret Life of Plants" covered the outcome of experiments detailing how emotional and intelligent plants are. When we interact with or even consume plants, we must keep in mind that we aren't just partaking dense substance but also a form of cosmic intelligence as the plants have been proven to have a life of their own in a much more complex manner than formerly believed. While our ancestors may have been familiar with the wisdom that plants inherently possess, the modern world experienced a recent phase of enlightenment regarding this. The plant kingdom has been shown to have its own set of neural networks and multifaceted communities beneath the soil. Plants have their own ways for dealing with toxins and low frequencies that appear to be more advanced than ours as humans. They have processes for differentiating between genes and families and even respond intelligently to sound patterns and music played around them. We have been underestimating them for way to long and now is the time to create a better relationship with them and to increase the amount of respect we have for them. There is so much more to learn about them and from them.

Organic vs. Biodynamic

Nowadays the word organic has be copy written and no longer seems to resonate with its original meaning. It is derived from the ancient word Arajun meaning to return or "the name of a circle". It means that something comes from the source and eventually goes back to it. Pharmaceutical companies and others with large enough pockets have been paying to get their genetically modified foods under the radar for years now. The stores can no longer be trusted because most of the large chains are being paid off. The only way to ensure that your food is organic is to grow it yourself. There are plenty of families who have preserved seeds for purchase and if that method is not one you trust then nature has its own formula. Consuming is not recommended during the process, but you can plant seeds in clean and healthy soil and replant the ones from the crops grown over a period of 4 to 5 years as nature restores the seeds integrity from any genetic alterations from chemicals sprayed or used in previous fields or gardens. The sunlight will destroy foreign substances in the genes of the plant over time. The hue of the seed will be a indicator of the improvements made over time. The carbon restoration will show up as a blacker or browner seed color as opposed to a pale or tan one. All original things start off with blackness or rely on blackness in order to be manifested.

The organic approach is ecologically sound and strives to replace an overly complex method with a commonsense approach which the ordinary farmer or gardener can relate to. Insects and many diseases are combated using nature's own remedies like ladybugs, trichogramma, praying mantises, garlic, pepper sprays, neem, etc. The goal is to produce healthy soil for health plants to be consumed by healthy animals and humans. Biodynamics is also ecologically sound but takes a much wider scope into account, including the sun, the phases of the moon, and subterranean features in efforts to understand the sum total of all their factors. Based on critical observation of nature, this approach calls for not allowing for things to run their natural course, but for intensifying certain natural process i.e., creating optimal animal populations, making special compost preparations, planting selected companion plants at times when specific constellations have the greatest influence on an environment, etc. It aids nature where she appears to be weak after centuries of abuse, short-cutting destructive processes, and using human compassion, kindness, and goodwill to make positive developments like planting hedges and building houses for birds, making pastures for bees, etc. Biodynamics can be used as a human service to the earth and its creatures as we strive to manifest balance. While both practices are commonly aimed at producing healthy food, we must understand that healthy food is not enough to change the world. What we do with the foods we consume is much more important.

Biodynamics can be summed up as putting our energy into supporting the good as opposed to fighting the bad. Low productivity, unwanted insects, and diseases are not the problem. They are the symptoms. Spraying bugs, using unnatural chemicals and other means of combating issues is treating the symptom, whereas doing things like nurturing the soil and improving our relationship with the land is solving the actual problem.

Pest Prevention
Aphid Wasps
Ladybird Beetles
Ladybugs
Lacewing Larvae
Mason Wasps
Assassin Bugs
Diatomaceous Earth
Neem Oil
Peppermint Spray

Every time we take a breath we recalibrate the body. The physical body is our personal portion of Mother Nature. She is always at work seeking balance and restoration. Our bodies as an extension of her are constantly doing everything in their power to maintain order as a holographic expression of nature's original agenda.

Section 11 Summary

Our Mother Earth is abundant and has everything we need to be healthy, happy, and divine. It is our duty to understand her, and most importantly, to take care of her. We only have one planet earth, and it is up to us to protect her at all costs.

Much of the unusual things we're experiencing in the world is a result of us abusing our planet from us polluting the waters and land, overusing natural resources, to us industrializing everything. We have not been working in harmony with the planet. Only bad things will happen if we continue down this path. Love this planet the way you love your human mama.

Your Diet

Ch.47: Choose Your Own Diet

We learn about new diets every year. Many people detox themselves to death from not understanding how the body works and from following trends online that may or may not pertain to them. Again, we are here to remind you that there are many different systems to address when attempting to restore our body and that everything is not for everybody. Depending on our cosmic and biological makeup, our body may require foods and activities that do not pertain to others around us. A sure way to get clear about what we need is to get a birth chart reading from a professional and seasoned astrologer. Our moon sign along with our 2nd house, 6th house, and 10th house placements are significant when it comes to the type of diets that are most ideal for us.

Types of Diets	Description
Standard American	Anything goes if it tastes good
Pescatarian	Fish is allowed in the diet
Vegetarian	Dairy is allowed in the diet
Vegan	No meat derived foods are allowed
Raw Food Vegan	Living and vibrant or dried foods only
Fruitarian	Only fruit is consumed
Breatharian	Only sunlight and air are consumed
Paleo	Foods obtained primarily by hunting and gathering
Ketogenic	Low carbs and high fat content to promote ketosis

Diets that contain large amounts of animal foods are associated with several chronic diseases not because meat is bad for us but because it is more of a challenge for us to break it down. Another contributor to the illusion of meat being bad is the fact that it is more differentiated than fruits and vegetables, which have more of an affinity to the undifferentiated state of substance that allows for all vibrations. The more differentiated or distinguished a food or animal is, the more energy must be used to break it down to integrate it and make it apart of the body. Remember that everything vibrates and some things are simply easier to deal with than others but ultimately all things can be broken down back into their least common denominators i.e. hydrogen, carbon, and oxygen whether it be thru natural biological processes or transmutation and the level of difficulty during this process is what calls for people to classify a food as healthy (easily broken down and conformed) or not healthy (hard to break down resulting in an accumulation until the substance is able to be addressed properly).

Consistency is just as important as the foods you choose to eat. How frequently one chooses to consume a particular food greatly influences the magnitude and effect of that food in their body. It is also important that we eat foods found and grown naturally in Mother Nature as opposed to processed foods so that we can consume and harmonize with the primordial forces of the universe in their original condition. When people choose to eat manufactured or processed foods, they are limiting their participation with the natural order of the universe. Refined foods do not supply the body with negative ions, which is one of our primary sources of fuel.

As we go through life prayerfully fulfilling our purpose on earth, bodily systems continue to do their jobs while we use up minerals and the benefits of consumed substances. We find ourselves feeling hungry when in fact this is the body communicating to us that we need water or nutrients. It is important to understand that the body is not hungry for the food itself but for the minerals contained within the foods we eat.

Foods and Supplements For High Vibratory Cells	
Vitamin A	Bitter Melon
All B Vitamins (Complex)	co-enzyme Q10
Vitamin C	Silica
Vitamin E	Cysteine
Vitamin K	Tocotrienols
Flavanoids	Lipoic Acid
Selenium	Long & Short Chain Essential Fatty Acids
EPA	DHA
Iron (From Plants)	Copper
Chondrus Crispus	Phytoplankton
Sea Buckthorn	Baobab
Lemons	Limes

These nutrients help to strengthen the integrity of our cells and to build our biochemical and vibration determined immune system responses. They also help to alkalize and oxygenate the body.

Vegan vs. Healthy

While veganism is highly recommended and especially so during cleansing processes, it is not mandatory for spiritual development or for the fulfilling of one's purpose. It is however a great dietary choice for those who need a thorough internal cleansing or those who are interested in optimization of the physical body which should not be confused with optimizing human potential or any of the more subtle bodies leading us back to the true self. When consuming what one might call a vegan diet it is important to not be fooled into thinking that meat substitutes and the modern commercial vegan options are means to returning the body back into its original state. To put the body in its most premium condition, it is necessary to separate the fad of veganism from the actual science of the body and what it requires of us. The fulfillment of one's purpose is much more important that his or her food selection. The diet at most is a means for nourishing and maintaining the physical instrument that we need to ultimately accomplish what we were born to do. Whatever you should end up choosing for yourself is perfectly fine and is solely up to you at the end of the day. Your value is not determined by what you put into your mouth but is measured by your contribution and service to the collective.

Eating in Season

Fresh cosmic fuel from the foods in season serves as a provider of up-to-date messages from the universe also referred to as light code transmissions. In the same way that iPhones require constant upgrades, we too are allowed to become enhanced and evolve with the universe around us. We are infinite beings constantly taking on different forms and arrangements with every inhale and exhale. We can essentially change in any manner of our liking so long as those changes honor the laws of the mind and human body (which are simple and allow for countless possibilities) but the most beneficial of the forms we can manifest are those where we are most in sync with the universe.

If one is interested in being more detailed with his or her eating in harmony with nature, they can study and practice what is referred to as the macrobiotic diet. It is currently practiced heavily in Asia but had its origin in ancient Africa just as with most things. This dietary practice has proven to extend the lives of its practitioners to lengths beyond the average person with normal eating habits.

Winter Areas To Address (Dec 20 thru March 20)
Kidneys
Bladder
Adrenals
Bones
Urinary Tract
Reproductive System

Spring Areas To Address (March 21 thru June 20)
Liver
Gallbladder
Joints and Tendons
Nervous System
Musculoskeletal System

Summer Areas To Address (June 21 thru Aug 20)
Heart
Small Intestines
Circulatory System
Blood

Late Summer Areas To Address (Aug 21 thru Sept 20)
Stomach
Spleen
Pancreas
Digestive System

Fall Areas To Address (Sept 21 thru Dec 19)
Lungs
Large Intestines
Skin
Respiratory System
Immune System

These particular dates are relevant for individuals living on the western hemisphere. If you live in another part of the world, be sure to use dates that correspond to the change of seasons on the part of the planet you domicile in.

Ch.48: Nutrients

In cooperation with sunlight, water, and fresh air, nutrients help us to sustain and maintain our physical bodies. Examples can be found all throughout this book but understand that they are essential for the production of and optimal human body. Eat as you please but be sure to balance the diet of your choice with proper nutrients.

Enzymes are a necessary nutrient that the body requires for peak immunity and optimal performance. Some of them are specifically dedicated to digestion and help us to break down substances called polymeric macromolecules into smaller forms that allow for us to absorb nutrients properly. The body was designed for food to be digested and moved through the alimentary canal within a twelve-hour window. The colon is literally the sewer system of the body. We should be having a bowel movement for every meal that we eat throughout the day. A sluggish and inactive colon and a fatty liver can cause the body to do a poor job of maintaining its oxidative metabolism. Living foods have an abundance of naturally occurring enzymes that assist us in preventing such a problem.

Bioavailability is the measure of a nutrients ability to cross the cell membrane in order to become assimilated with our cells. Enzymes disassemble colloids of a nutrient, increasing its surface are, resulting in an enormous maximizing of its bioavailability.

Nutrients like co-enzyme Q10 help us to fuel each cell's super rich energy compound known as Adenosine Triphosphate or ATP. Cells use ATP for 95% of their energy requirements.

More on Adenosine Triphosphate or ATP

The condition in the cell is influenced by the ionization of potassium, sodium, calcium, magnesium, and ATP. The function of ATP is then regulated by an enzyme ATP-ase, which is sensitive to radiation and light and helps with photosynthesis and other light-based transductions. By using ATP as its energy source, the neuron membranes in our body can pump sodium ions out of the cell as fast as they diffuse inward through the cell wall to maintain a balance of electrical charge. This fine balance allows cells to become extremely sensitive to small electrical stimuli in their external environment.

Alkalinity and Acidity

Alkalinity causes a current and we have energy. When the battery is too acidic, our spare electrons are expended. The body becomes low in energy and degeneration begins. The cause of much illness in the modern so-called civilized world is due to the premature degradation of tissue (via extreme acidity) and the body system thru decomposition by bacteria, mold, fungus, and yeast. Eating fresh fruit and vegetables which are easily digested on the other hand, creates good internal hygiene, resulting in an environment for clean and healthy blood. Keeping blood and body tissue at a proper pH keeps premature death at bay and makes the difference between vitality and death. This is one of the secrets of an alkaline body.

When our bodies are alkaline, we have spare electrons and having spare electrons equals having longer life. Unsaturated fats are important in biology because they supply the body with an abundance of spare electrons.

Cysteine is a sulfur bearing amino acid that has a positive electric charge. It can be found in nuts and can make unsaturated plant fates soluble.

Ch.49: A Healthier You

Decongest: Breakdown and purge heavy areas that need to be loosened up to prepare for an effective detox. Exercise and foods like haritaki fruit or citrus fruits are excellent options for this first phase. (This is also the time to clean your home, workspaces, and your environments. Uncluttering and organizing are useful practices as well.)

Detox: Remove toxins with chlorophyll rich plants and drinks. The body strives to break what it can down into a liquid form. Green drinks are recommended over an increase in green leafy vegetables even though the latter is an effective choice when juices are not an option. (Forgive and release toxicity from subtle areas via old emotions like worry, fear, grief, depression, etc.)

Cleanse: After the toxins are removed, it is important to go and clean up the cells from the effects of the poisons that were just removed. Fruits are hands down the greatest cellular cleansers on the planet. Dark and tropical fruits are the most efficient at cleansing.

Nourish: Re-mineralizing and revitalizing the cells is key for conducting, storing, and housing different forms of light. Sea moss and other foods with a plethora of minerals like phytoplankton are ideal during this phase. (Surround yourself with individuals who cater better to your overall sense of wellbeing.)

Polish: Even though we will continue to run into challenges during our experience on Earth, performing purification methods monthly or during each season will significantly decrease the possibility and potential of reoccurring issues. (Stay in the Sun and around large bodies of water as much as humanly possible!)

Formula One for Cancer Elimination and Cellular Cleansing
1 part Dandelion Root
1 part Yellow Dock Root
1 part Wild Indigo
2 Parts Turmeric
1 part Venus Fly Trap
1 part Mistletoe
1 part Astragalus
1 part Blue Vervain
¼ part Cordyceps

Formula Two for Cancer Elimination and Cellular Cleansing
1 part Mandrake
1 part Red Clover
1 part Blessed Thistle
2 Parts Chondrus Crispus
1 part Heal-All
1 part Blue Violet
1 part Black Walnut
1 part Blue Vervain
2 parts St. John's wort

Formula Three for Cancer Elimination and Cellular Cleansing
1 part Peppermint
1 part Yellow Dock Root
1 part Bitter Melon
2 Parts Trumpet Creeper Root
1 part Celandine
1 part Dulse
1 part Mimosa Bark
1 part Blue Vervain
1 part Wormwood

Try these herbs on a 21-60 day schedule while resting at least 2-3 days out of the week so that the cells are not overworked during the cleansing process

A Holistic Approach

Just as the zodiacal wheel continues in a full circle, true health requires of us to address ourselves holistically and not just physically. Our actions and attention need to be spread around the full spectrum of life. The signs correspond to their respective systems in the body while the house rule the various departments in our life i.e. our personal space, our home, our workplace, etc. The first six houses of our chart deals with our individual makeup and what we bring to any given situation. The seventh through twelfth houses deal more with how we function in the world outside of self.

1st House Ruled (Natural Home to Aries)

The first house deals with our general health, the physical status of the body and its physiological needs. In particular, the first house deals with health shortly after birth and the environment that we grow up in. This house is also referred to as the ascendant and represents the moment we are born. It is also associated with health conditions related to the head i.e. issues with the teeth, eyes, acne, or mental diseases.

2nd House (Natural Home to Taurus)

The second house deals with our finances, our tastes and food preferences, our self-esteem and sense of self worth, and our value system in general. It reveals to us our priorities and our feelings regarding our sensations and our possessions.

3rd House (Natural Home to Gemini)

The third house represents our siblings, personal studies, mental activities, short travels and shines a light on issues or matters pertaining to our breathing or the respiratory system in general.

4th House (natural Home to Cancer)

The fourth house represents our home, our personal environment, the relationship we have with our parents, and the way that we nurture ourselves. It can also shine a light on issues or matters dealing with our overall immunity and the condition of our lymphatic system.

5th House (Natural Home to Leo)

The fifth house represents the way that we promote ourselves to the rest of the world. It shines a light on the ways that we choose to love and deals with pleasurable emotions. Many astrologers also tend to associate the fifth house with children and how we interact with the youth. It also reveals issues or matters concerned with our blood and the circulatory system.

6th House (Natural Home to Virgo)

The sixth house represents different sicknesses that we may be prone to especially those concerning the gastrointestinal tract. It represents the areas that we may offer the best services in to benefit humanity. It corresponds with our employees if we have them, our personal craft or work in general, our hygiene, our dietary preference and matters associated with the solar plexus.

7th House (Natural Home to Libra)

The seventh house generally relates to people we consult on a one to one basis. In medical astrology this house represents our relationship with doctors, nutritionists, astrologers, psychologists, and anyone who is consulted for our health problems. It also represents our marriages, contracts, lawsuits, public dealings and open enemies. The seventh house reveals issues or matters involving the kidneys and our excretory system in general.

8th *House (Natural Home to Scorpio)*

The eighth house is referred to by many astrologers as the house of death and resonates with all matters connected to the dead but we can also conclude that this house corresponds with areas in life that we transmute circumstances or energy in. Death can also refer to habits, states of consciousness, relationships, diseases etc. The ninth house reveals issues or matters involving our reproductive health.

9th *House (Natural Home to Sagittarius)*

The ninth house corresponds with long distance relationships, foreign lands, and places that are far from where we were born. It also vibrates with our higher levels of learning or wisdom pertaining to our spiritual matters i.e. dreams, spiritual powers, and visions. The ninth house shines a light on issues or matters pertaining to our muscular system.

10th House (Natural Home to Capricorn)

The tenth house governs our profession in life, promotions of any sort, our employer, the affairs of the land we live on or the government we participate with. It also shines a light on issues or matters pertaining to our skeletal system.

11th House (Natural Home to Aquarius)

The eleventh house deals with our friends and associates. It governs the channels that energy moves about in our body and sheds light on our humanitarian efforts or our spirit of altruism.

12th House (Natural Home to Pisces)

The twelfth house deals with our suffering and the lessons we can learn from it. It reveals our secret problems, our secret enemies and our interactions with hospitals. Our apparent limitations and self-undoing is done here as we polish and improve ourselves. Our inner world resonates with this house and can either cause of anguish or lead us in the best direction if we learn from the pressures of the problems we face. The twelfth house also reveals matters involving the integumentary system.

We know from many religious doctrines that we are made in the image and likeness of our creator. The functions and rulership of the houses of the zodiac reveal to us how wholesome and balanced our creator is.

Healthy Essentials
Healthy Mitochondria
Great Immunity
T Cell Production
Free Flowing Blood and Lymph
Structured or EZ Water
Exercise via Calisthenics and Isometrics
Healthy Microbiome
High Frequency Internal Vibrations

Hot To Decrease Your Energy Levels
Stress
Lack of sunlight
Denatured foods
Dehydration
Inconsistent sleeping patterns or lack of sleep
Spending too much time indoors
Stagnation
Too much carbon dioxide
Cluttered spaces
Confusion
Fear

How To Increase Your Energy Levels
Productive meditation sessions
Sunlight exposure
Living foods
Super hydration
Consistent sleeping patterns
Spending time with Mother Nature
Exercise
Fresh oxygen
Organization
Mental clarity

Look at yourself like a lifelong project and determine how you will arrange and utilize the light responsible for the structure and functioning of our universe. There is work to be accomplished in and around us everyday.

Section 12 Summary

An explosive revelation of this section is veganism does not equal healthy. One thing that was real about the beginning of our pandemic was COVID-19 did not discriminate against anyone, vegans included. Right along with the carnivores, obese, drug abusers, or anyone that society has deemed unhealthy, were also vegetarians and vegans, folks who are assumed to be healthier than everyone else. While we can argue that a plant-based life has many benefits and could present a better quality of life for us, vegetarianism and veganism is not the only route towards optimal health.

Keeping in mind that the theme in this work is a healthier spirit, mind, and body means your diet either enhances your spiritual and mental health or lowers it. Another way to wording this is good food brings your vibration higher while bad food lowers it. Always have this in the back of your mind when picking your diet.

Regardless of whether you are eating plants or animals, make sure you are avoiding over-processed or fake food at all costs. If there's an enemy in the food realm, it is the stuff that's created in a factory or lab. Eat real foods as much as possible and you will be much better off.

Defense

Ch.50: On Immunity

T-Cells, which are a major contributor to our immune system, recognize antigens and foreign substances by means of proteins in their cell membranes called T- cell receptors. These T-cell receptors require a class of immune proteins called MHCs to bind to foreign protein in our body. MHC is short for major histocompatibility complex, which is a group of genes that code for proteins found on the surface of cells. T-cells and NK lymphocyte cells are a part of our acquired immune system. Antibodies produced by B-cells in our blood plasma, can recognize foreign proteins like antigens. Our naturally occurring antibodies specifically bind to antigens, labeling this debris for it to be evacuated from the body or for its structure to be disassembled.

Physical health depends on us maintaining the proper internal and external hygiene. Our ancient chemical/bioelectrical-mediated immunity, along with four types of proteins i.e. antibodies, T-cell receptors, MHC, and RAG proteins keep our internal terrain hygienic and well ordered. In a clean body, our immune system is educated as to what is self and what is other than self. In this way, dendritic cells, which are imbedded in between cells, sample the terrain to identify toxins and alert immune cells. In an immune compromised body, dendritic cells do not expose themselves and as a result of this immune cells are not informed and instructed to respond properly.

Initiating great hygiene is one thing but sustaining proper internal hygiene requires having exceptional physical and biochemical protective mechanism factors. Some examples of these are the skin, our digestive juices, inflammatory and healing responses, and different types of cells that are capable of disassembling foreign bacteria and tumors. All these factors are specific morphology responses effected to ensure that we can maintain cell homeostasis. Thyroid tissue is more alkaline than the brain and plays an essential role in our overall immunity. The thyroid and endocrine functions are often taxed when the body uses its immunity to respond to foreign protein, thus reinforcing the need for restoration of these vital systems. Immune complexes consist of 9 primary proteins involving 27 known sub-proteins, of which 22 are enzymes. These complexes are a part of the immune cells ability to neutralize antigens and waste. Sweating is also one of the best ways to release toxins and waste from our body and it helps to balance our pH by excreting L-actic acid.

L. Salivarius, cultured from human breast milk colostrums, is a friendly bacterium that disassembles unwanted substances from the body. We are supposed to get our life's supply of colostrum in the first few days of life from our mother's breast. We highly encourage breast-feeding as opposed to the fad of using formula. Remaining hydrated is of the utmost importance during this time.

Immune System Contributors
Melanin
Lymphatic Fluids
Lymph Nodes and Vessels
Immune Cells
Bone Marrow
Thymus Gland
Sleen
Physical Barriers

Memory cells are created by T and B cells so that the body remembers specific invaders. The immune memory is developed so stronger, more efficient responses can be initiated when necessary.

Drink, Breath, Reset

Ch.51: You Are Not Wet Enough

We know that the body is 99.9% water but often times we forget that everything in it is made up of water as well. The brain is composed of 80-90% water as it sits in a basin of water to remain hydrated. Our lymphatic system is made entirely of water and our blood is 80-95% water. Our heart is about 85% water as it houses the body's largest magnetic field, and our lungs expand and contract next to it also being composed of the same amount. Even our bones are composed of about 25-30% water and our muscles about 90%. Our kidneys are made up of about 80% water while our liver is just a tad bit denser falling right behind that percentage at about 75% water. There is no way to get around it. This should not be a surprise since we are essentially light beings and water is known to be a super conductor of light and electricity, which is only a lesser degree of light. Even though our bodies are made of water, we still need to replace it daily since all our activities require it whether it is something as simple as walking or talking. If we are to propel ourselves towards a healthier state of being, hydration is necessary and cannot be substituted, as it is essential for everything else to function correctly.

Water and lymph behave more like gas than a liquid inside us. They penetrate right through us, even through the dentin in our teeth. It has countless properties and scientists are still discovering ways to benefits from it to this day. It gets lighter as it becomes more solid as seen when ice floats at the top of a glass of water or juice. Water is also the most important solvent on our planet and is known to be a living substance. It is so alive that the hydrogen atoms slip from one end of the oxygen atom to the other continuously in a synchronized manner. The water inside of our blood is supremely structured as the water molecules unite to make hexagonal and pentagonal shapes.

We have mentioned that water is essential for all life on Earth however many of us have not grasped that the older we get, the more dehydrated we become. One of the best ways to combat this problem is to structure the water in our body so that it becomes more gel like than liquid. EZ water or exclusion zone water is the term for this. EZ water pushes everything outside of the structured portion that is detrimental to the cell and scientists have discovered that when light shines on water, the EZ water or exclusion zone is expanded. This EZ water has been shown to have a negative charge that repels anything with a positive charge. The human cell can maintain its most optimal form resulting in the highest amounts of energy when it is composed of EZ water. While food is an excellent means of acquiring energy, both water and light are simpler sources and work wonders in our body when they complement each other. Out of all our food options, fruits are the best example of an edible form of exclusion zone water. Fruit is literally organized and structured water vibrating at a particular rate revealing to us its color. The color then reveals to us the type of nutrients dominating the molecular configuration of the fruit. This exclusion zone water has been coined "the fourth phase of water" and has been shown to be one of the healthiest forms of water for us to consume.

EZ or Structured Water Explained

Water is layered when it is bound to protein. The first layer is fixed more to the protein substances. The layer furthest out is referred to as bulk water while the layer in between is titled as the interface layer. Enzymes are active inside the interface layer. This water has a lower freezing point at negative ten degrees Celsius. Sixty-four percent of this interface layer is mainly hexagonal shaped water structure like what we see with snowflakes. The interface layer is consequently the best layer of water for plankton and algae to grow in because it is so highly structured. This structure is responsible for the cohesion and the levels of intelligence found in these plants as well.

Healthy body tissue has the structured interface layer of water, while distorted tissue lacks it. Hexagonal formed water structure is found near ionized calcium. Ionization is an activity that can occur naturally inside of water, like with electrolytes for example. Ionization occurs in the body when oxygen and hydrogen atoms gain or lose electrons, making them electrically and magnetically charged which results in greater levels of chemical activities. Ionized water splits in half. One of these halves is the H+ ion (acid) and the other is the hydroxyl ion OH- (alkaline). The concentration of these two ions brings about enzyme homeostasis and life, as we know it.

Alkaline Forming Elements	Acid forming Elements
Potassium (K)	Silica (Si)
Sodium (Na)	Sulfur (S)
Calcium (Ca)	Phosphorus (P)
Magnesium (Mg)	Chlorine (Ch)
Iron (Fe)	Iodine (I)

Ch.52: Breathing Is Fundamental

Breathing is hands down one of the most important acid/alkaline buffers. The alveoli in our lungs are designed to maintain excellent oxidative metabolism by balancing the oxygen and carbon dioxide ratio in our body. Relaxed, quiet, and calm breathing causes the alveoli to continuously trap carbon dioxide-causing carbonic acid, which raises the acidity of the erythrocytes or red blood cells and brings about healthy oxygenation throughout the whole body. Our blood has a profound ability to release its oxygen which otherwise would result in free radicals and active oxygen to cause sedimentation and the coagulation of substances in our connective tissue that causes a hardening of that connective tissue and vascular and neural tissue contraction as well as issues like sclerosis.

Breathing brings life to the cells. Robust deep breathing oxygenates our entire bodily system, which is extremely significant for the brain. Proper breath and other habits involving our internal and external hygiene, allows for body fluids to functionally hydrate our cells. If our body remains hydrated, our connective tissue will maintain a youthful essence. Hydrated cells which can be many times as hydrated as dehydrated ones give a person a youthful glowing appearance.

Respiratory System Components
Nose
Trachea
Bronchi
Lungs
Diaphragm
Secondary Respiratory Muscles

Oxygen is a critical component of most of our cellular functions in the body. Breathwork has been shown to improve the quality of our immune system, circulatory system, autonomic nervous system, and various mental disorders.

Secondary respiratory muscles include the scalenes, pectorals, external intercostals and the sternocleidomastoid.

Ch.53: On Fasting

To fast simply means to abstain from something and this can be applied to people, places, or things but here in this discussion we are referring to foods. Our body strives to break our meals down into a liquid form in order for the nutrients in our food to be absorbed into the walls of our intestines. Juicing fruits and vegetables works to free the body from having to do excess work as it provides clean liquid nutrition directly into our cells. When the digestive tract is no longer using its energy to breakdown foods, the body can use its energy to regenerate and rebalance the body back into a more optimal and wholesome state. When we fast for long enough the body uses a method called autophagy where it discards damaged and detrimental cells to kick start the rejuvenation process. The active molecules in this process are claw like and pull toxins out of our cells. Autophagy also allows for chelation in the body. This results in improved absorption when we choose to return to eating regular again.

Fasting also increases our redox potential, which results in an increase of voltage and electrical potential in our body. It allows for our cells to perform in a different manner than normal since they are typically busy responding to us eating various amounts of meals throughout the day. They begin to focus on restorative functions as opposed to their usual activities. From just three days of fasting, we can relax the body enough to reset our immune systems. This is actually an ancient habit to practice each month, or one could take a break from their usual eating routines every season in order to give the body a chance to breathe and recalibrate. If a monthly practice is chosen, the moon will serve as an excellent tool for timing as it is the origin of how we determine a month anyway.

Be sure to respect graduality as you transition back into you normal eating habits after fasting. If you have been consuming nothing but water and juice, then you may want to consider sticking to fruits for a few days and then fresh greenery in the days following. If you rush back into eating flesh or heavy meals on your first day after fasting, you may experience uncomfortable feelings, headaches, or even feel as though your body has come to a halt for a while because you have shocked your body. A gradual transition back into normal eating is best since we are creatures of habit and work off rhythms and vibration. Make it a point to refrain from mental and social activities in addition to abstinence from poor foods to ensure the best results.

Vegan Food Breakdown

Sunlight and Structured water (25%)

Algae and Seaweed (10%)

Herbs and Sprouts (10%)

Nuts and Seeds (5%)

Fruits and Vegetables (25%)

Leafy Greenery and Ancient Grains (25%)

Non-Vegan Food Breakdown

Sunlight and Water (25%)

Vitamin and Mineral Supplements (5%)

Meat, Fish and Dairy (10%)

Grains and Cereals (10%)

Fruits and Vegetables (40%)

Breads, Cereals, and Pastas (10%)

Eat For Your Haplotype

All plants have a specific range of vibration according to their mineral composition and the part of the planet in which they are grown. All plants are indigenous to certain areas on our planet and even though they can be transplanted and shared with other parts of the world, they grow best and become most potent in those areas that they are natural grown in. Even though Dr. Sebi is most famous for promoting an alkaline diet, those who walked and talked with him personally understood that to be only the portion that most people were able to digest at the time. He stressed to those with minds capable of understanding the importance of eating according to our genetic make up or more appropriately stated, according to our haplotype. An easy way of comprehending this is to eat according to the genes that we inherited from our parents. Blood types are trendy to go by in this day and age but do us no good in the long run since they can be altered over time thru diet and environments. It should be understood by now that red blood cells are the same essentially and that the amount and kind of antigens is what distinguishes the different types of blood that we are familiar with today i.e. A, B, AB, O, and so on. While genetics can be influenced in a variety of ways, they can only be altered so much due to the intense impact that our lineage has on us. The following is a list of plants and their places of origin so we can get an idea of what it means to consume foods from where you or your family are native to. By all means enjoy your human experience and eat what you please but be sure to make room in your diet to honor the vibrations that are responsible for getting you to where you are now.

Recommended Food Lists

The following list **(List A)** is more relevant when the Earth's magnetic field is optimal. If this is not the case then we cannot expect Mother Nature to produce her most premium foods. Consuming the Sun is primary when it comes to nutrition and the maintenance of the physical body. The Sun is in fact the manufacturer of the physical body. Now we can see why there is an alteration in the outcome of foods when the Earth's relationship with the Sun is altered. We have put together a Food List to cater to you in that altered state as well. **(See List B)**

List A: A High Frequency Food List:

Prayer (Concentrated thought) and Meditation (Listening for instructions/guidance)

Sunlight

Fresh Air

Structured water

Phytoplankton

Sea moss

Blur-Green Algae

Other Red Algae

Sea Vegetables (i.e. Kelp, Wakame, Arame, Nori, Dulse, etc.)

Camu Camu Berries

Blueberries

Blackberries

Raspberries

Dark Hued Mulberries

Cherries

Watermelons

Dates

Tamarind

Mandarin

Lemons

Limes

Citrons

Nettle

Hemp

Cilantro

Parsley

Burdock

Yellow Dock

Blue Vervain

Clove

Black walnut

Wormwood

Cleavers

Hydrangea

Dandelion Plantain

Coriander

List B: Premium Survival Food List:

Clear and Capable Mind

Sunlight

Fresh Air (Oxygen)

Structured Water

Dried Fruit

Fish

Deer

Lamb

Alligator or Crocodile

Birds

Goats

Milk Thistle (Liver repair)

Clove (Parasite killer)

Hemp (A plethora of uses spanning from clothes to the construction of buildings)

African Pygeum Bark (Energy and Endurance)

Energy Bars (These can be prepared using hemp seeds, dates, dried cranberries, raw honey, pumpkin seeds, sunflower seeds, and walnuts)

Black Seeds (For sustained energy and nutrients)

The goal is to make sure we have the plants available to help repair any internal system or external part of the body.

Non-Perishable Foods

(Strive to gather at least 2-3 months worth of foods per person and ideally a year worth of these recommendations)

1. Pure Raw Honey

2. Black or wild rice

3. Dried beans or lentils

4. Nut butters like cashew or

5. Sunflower or pumpkin seeds

6. Dried fruit

7. Dried herbs

8. Dried chili peppers

9. Ancient grains

10. Dried soup mixes

11. Dried sea vegetables

12. Granola bars or cereal

DIY Energy Examples

Wood burning stove

Propane to feed a propane stove

Gasoline generator

Solar cells

Deep cycle batteries

Power inverters

Solar Panels

Power Generating Wind Mills

Power generating playgrounds

Energy diversity is extremely important and will eventually be necessary for survival.

For Colored Folks Only

Ch.54: Challenges to Overcome in the Black and Brown Communities

Our black and brown communities are dealing with double sided problems that we also have the best solutions to. We as a people are suffering from unhealthy bodies and minds and also poverty along with its corresponding effects. Some of the biggest hindrances to our liberation are our lack of both self-control and unity. As we become more self-aware we will see an increase of love for ourselves and those who share our divinely endowed qualities and characteristics. Our perception of self plays such a critical role in our progress during these times that we must get clear about it as we make and keep it a priority.

The Illusion of White Supremacy

This system is designed to keep us ignorant when it comes to our history and the powers that we are naturally endowed with. It drains people of their time and energy while they are in a constant state of trying to catch back up and most people never succeed. It leaches on people and their energy in order to maintain its image of being a necessity while in reality it is the reason that people have the problem of needing anything in the first place. Abundance is our natural inheritance and we have the opportunity each day to instruct the universe when it comes to how much of that abundance is allowed to flow thru us. (Jupiter)

On The Medical industry

The so-called father of modern biology is said to be Thomas Rivers who was funded by David Rockefeller. He and his colleagues manipulated the medical industry in order to get allopathic doctors to promote the idea of using poisons to kill germs. The "contagion myth" has caused many unnecessary deaths and problems in society due to people's ignorance and lack of self-accountability. Nowadays we are benefiting from a growing number of people who are addressing things at the causal level which will result in the elimination of problems that we tend to struggle with downstream from there.

Things To Take Into Consideration When Striving To Heal Our People

Our *level of self-awareness* directly influences our nervous system and indirectly impacts all the remaining systems in the human body.

Our *genetics* should be taken into consideration and it should be understood that the more we dishonor them with practices foreign to our own, the more prone we will be to disease states from misalignment.

Our *diets* are relevant because they play a huge role when it comes to our energy consumption and the quality of fuel we run on. Eating foods that are manmade and full of chemical additives, antibiotics, pesticides, etc. will slowly but surely make the body other than what it is intended to be.

Emotional and *mental stress* from anger, fear, grief, and other low vibratory feelings weaken the immune and nervous systems causing stunted immune response and other physical disorders.

Environmental pollution from the air, water, and soil contribute to disorders ranging from allergies to full blown cancer. This is especially true in cities with factories and high automobile activity.

Unnecessary vaccinations and *antibiotics* can cause the body to be altered even at a genetic level. Both of these when used inappropriately disrupt the balance of the body and promote a variety of maladies like ear infections, to food allergies, and immune suppression.

Extremely low frequencies also known as ELFs from computers, cell phones, televisions, electrical appliances, microwaves, etc. can induce chronic stress, stunted or deformed cell growth and division, neurochemical and genetic alterations, altered hormone production, tumor growth, and even viral outrage.

Ch.55: Bonus Portion

On Age Reversal

Various religious texts speak of people living up until around a thousand years old. Our modern day habits and practices are so far away from the original ways of humanity that we expect for people to only live up until around 60 or 70 years old and their lives are planned according to these low expectations. The truth is that there is not limit to the human being other than the one that is self imposed or the one set in place by his or her stellar influences.

Research the life of Li Ching-Yuen who is recorded as living from 1677-1933 making him 256 years old when he transitioned.

In order to reverse or stunt the aging process, we must eliminate the poor habits that speed up and promote the process in the first place. All of us will die eventually but in the meantime we have the option of maximizing our human experience. With a small amount of tweaks in the right places we can cause a shift and increase our youthfulness by the day. Wake up to a glass of water each day and remain hydrated throughout the day in order to break down foods and combat disease phenomena. Constantly cleansing throughout the year is also a sure way to get rid of undesirable substances in our body. The longer toxins remain in the body the more harmful they become as they are fed by low frequency environments, dehydration, and unnatural foods. Eat or juice a lemon or a few key limes after hydrating in the morning to stimulate the detoxification of the kidneys and the liver.

Be sure to not stuff the stomach with too many meals throughout the day and honor the horary rhythms in order to achieve the greatest state of balance. We absorb the nutrients from foods the best between 1pm and 3pm, as the small intestine is the most active during these hours. Notice the intermitted fasting becoming more popular by the years due to the fact that the digestive tract rest and slows its vibrations down around 7pm. Our last meal should be eaten before then. When cooking meals, strive to stick with avocado oil, coconut oil, and olive oils only for a balanced omega 3 and omega 6 balance. Consume real foods meaning fruits with seeds or real meats if you eat flesh as all real fruits and vegetables have a natural magnetic field and a spin orientation that matches the spin cycles found in our cells. Genetically modified foods have an opposing spin that creates discord and imbalances in the body. Rest as much as possible and strive to match your sleep cycle with the hours that the sun is not visible.

Telomeres are found at the end our chromosomes and are significant due to the fact that they serve as a means to measure how youthful or how aged we are biologically. They tend to get shorter each time a cell copies itself but the essential portions of the DNA remain intact. Telomeres can be described as the aging clock in our cells but can be altered via consciousness and food choices.

Resveratrol significantly increases telomere activity by improving the expression of the catalytic subunit of what is called human telomerase reverse transcriptase or hTRET. Resveratrol is a type of natural phenol and a phytoalexin produced by certain plants when they are under stress or injured. This is another display of how intelligent and misunderstood the plant kingdom is. Resveratrol can be found in foods like blueberries, raspberries, and mulberries.

*Our body's endocrine system provides a variety of information substances that are key to age reversal.

Youthfulness is indicative of potential and is not subject to ones chronological age. It is also important to note that our chronological age is completely different than our biological age. The former tell us how many times the earth has been around the sun since we've been born while the other reveals to us the condition that we are in with the standard being our youthful charged and hydrated state.

On Sleep

People who insure that they get adequate amounts of sleep at night are shown to have improved memory, attention spans, and learning capacity. On the other hand, those who deprive themselves of sleep are more prone to suffer from mental issues like ADHD, depression, bipolar disorder, schizophrenia, anxiety, and weaker immune systems. The National Sleep Foundation recommends that adults get between 7-8 hours of sleep at night but of course everyone is different and requires regeneration only to the degree that energy is expended and repairs are needed. Meditating in the morning after gratitude and hydration can be an easy way to remain conscious of how much rest you need by being present and paying attention to your energy levels and analyzing how you feel in your mind and body. Darkness and a quiet environment are extremely helpful when striving to get a good nights rest. Our brains release the sleep hormone melatonin as a result of being in complete darkness or extremely low levels of sunlight or artificial light. Avoiding electronic devices like phones and computers for at least an hour or two before resting can allow one to tap into the natural rhythms in the area as opposed to them being interfered with by placing your attention and thus your neurons on things that are of a lesser vibration resulting in consequences that correspond to the lack of harmony created. Our circadian rhythm is attuned to the Earth's natural day/night cycles where the only real lights in existence are those of the stars and what is reflected by the moon. Keep in mind that rest is short for restoration and sleeping not only makes us feel recharged in the morning but also allows for us to recalibrate and correct our relationship with the universe and its natural forces.

Chymotrypsin digests protein and is produced by the pancreas. Chymotrypsin is made during sleep when the body is restful and naturally digests trophoblastic cells. Melatonin helps our body move into an alkaline state as we sleep and regenerate. While we sleep, anabolic steroids are released to help restore and build up the body. We also tend to breathe slower while sleep and slowed breathing alkalizes the body. Discoveries are still being made today in regards to how impactful melatonin is in the human body.

Sleep is how we regenerate and is a means of rebalancing the body and mind so that we are more aligned with the universe around us.

Social Relationships and Health

Throughout the majority of the time that we have been in existence, people have been recorded as living in indigenous self sustained communities of a tribal nature that thrived as abundance made itself known through their constant success and contributions to our modern world. In our ancient communities people supported one another in all walks of life and considered the condition of the world as it was handed down to the next generation. Any detriment or benefit to an individual was considered a detriment or benefit to the collective. As a result of capitalism and other material first societies however, this power in the people based lifestyle has become inverted, giving rise to the illusion of separateness and the mindset that makes one believe that he or she should only work for the good of themselves while neglecting the happiness and prosperity of others. This type of thinking causes people to miss out on the love and mind blowing experiences that can be achieved from healthy relationships with others. Lacking healthy social relationships is not only a lonely form of existence but can lead to depression, anxiety, and feelings of disconnection from the wholesome nature of the universe. Seeking out and finding meaningful relationships in life that support your own personal growth while reciprocating that beneficial energy back to others can help both parties in almost any aspect of life. By all means be mindful of how you spend your time and energy with others but also definitely make it a point to find those individuals that you can create the best chemistry with so you that you all can contribute to the collective in more impactful and significant ways together. Our ancient but wisdom filled ways are necessary now more than ever and it is up to us to usher them back into our realities.

Remember how atoms work together to form molecules and molecules work together to form cells and so on until we see a fully developed human being. If we were to simply look inside of ourselves, we could learn a lot about how to commune and exchange with things outside of self. Inside us things work in concert with one and another as opposed to outside of ourselves where we fight and war with each other. In many urban areas, there are individuals who don't even know the names of their next-door neighbors. The concept and practice of coherence must be reintroduced into our communities if we are to stick around to witness the unification and success of our people on the planet at this time. Our neighbors and village members can be viewed as potential collaborations or a means of transforming or amplifying your personal contribution to humanity. When we learn to work in harmony with one another we will then see how fast and much we can cause change in this world of reflections and physicality.

The health and vitality of the women in your community is an excellent means of measuring the potential and power of the people that live there.

Holistic Learning vs. Fragmented Schooling

The purpose of education supposedly is to facilitate the development of a mature mind. We however live in a world where the educational systems are designed to usher the student into a capitalistic society so that their learning revolves around the success of the companies and businesses that they hope to be hired into as opposed to learning about crafts and talents that could possibly benefit the world and humanity in general. The students for the most part learn very little about themselves and some learn nothing at all in regards to their existence or how to function in this universe. This creates a whole set of problems as the lack of knowledge concerning the self results in a series of detrimental choices and actions that could have been avoided had the person been made aware of his or her make up and their relationship with things and phenomena outside of self. This is where we draw the line though and this is one of the many reasons why a book of this caliber was necessary at this time.

Wisdom, liberation and transcendence are forms of extraction. Gold is an excellent example of this as it is so fundamental that it cannot be purified and can only be extracted from rock or other substances that surround it. Likewise the truth is always present and can only be covered or surrounded by things. It can never be altered and always exists as a prerequisite for all other things. It is fundamental and alignment with it dissolves illusions and disperses falsehoods. The point of bringing this up is to show that all the answers that we need to usher in the inevitable new reality being manifested on the planet at this time are already in existence and we simply need to uncover them and implement them. By living and operating in truth we are able to both harmonize and coexist in the best way with other people and the universe outside of us.

Make sure that what you learn while studying yourself helps to improve your understanding. Do not get caught up in memorizing information if you are not going to seek out an understanding of it.

Ch.56: A Healthy Vocabulary

Absolute entails all things including that which we deem infinite. There is nothing in existence that is not apart of the absolute. This feature of the creator allows for all possibilities and true health entails acknowledging it as our home before it becomes differentiated into its many components.

Breathing is our primary method of exchanging energy with the universe outside of our personal body. It is essential to all biological activities and serves as a prerequisite for energy production.

Balance is required for true health to be experienced. An unbalanced body will inevitably result in some form of disease until the substance or habit responsible is removed.

Centered and poised states can be achieved after balance is reached. Finding our center allows for us to be aware of ourselves completely.

Creativity is a divinely endowed gift from the creator that allows for us to participate in the creation process as eternity unfolds.

Development takes place whether we acknowledge it or not. It will always be in direct proportion to the manner in which we deal with the challenges presented to us in life.

Destiny is essentially determined by the thoughts we choose to think. We can eat and drink and observe as these things effect us but it is our thinking that brings us to those experiences and all others. By becoming more cautious of the thoughts we choose to entertain we can steer ourselves in more desirable directions as we navigate throughout our lives.

Excellence is what distinguishes a select few from the masses however it is slowly but surely becoming a requirement for survival as we transition between paradigms.

Equilibrium is found after each and every choice we make whether it is a physical or mental one. We are altering our condition with every breath, thought, and action. Each bite or sip we tap is meaningful when it comes to determining our outcomes.

Fasting is an ancient method whereby we can eliminate any and all things that create discomfort or disease in us. It simply means to abstain from and is a priceless practice to use for conquering addictions, diets, habits and undesirable circumstances.

Food is anything that interfaces with the body and mind. This includes substances that are edible, sounds that enter into our environments and any forms of energy that penetrate into our personal magnetic field.

Goals are helpful especially when it comes to mental orientation as they can be used to differentiate between actions in alignment with our purpose and distractions that steer us away from what we intend to manifest.

Healing is simply the process of returning back to our original state. It is a lot simpler than we make it out to be.

Haplotype is derived from the words haploid and genotype. It biologically defines our lineage and what we should begin to honor via our diet and lifestyle when striving to achieve optimal levels of health. Be sure to include foods in your diet that are indigenous to areas your ancestors frequented.

Inertia in its original meaning refers to the undisturbed and undifferentiated state of ether. Just as free energy is becoming popular from the technology able to tap into it, we too have the ability to access it before it is altered in any way. By being still and silencing our voices and minds we make it easier to tap into this primal state at any given time.

Inner Action is the true and relevant work we must consciously perform in our personal lives. This consists of using our awareness to make the necessary changes within ourselves as we make our daily exchanges with the universe around us. Learning, negating, and realizing among other things are examples of this.

Juxtaposition is when two elements are placed close together or side by side creating contrast or comparison between the two. In this text we employ the reader to consider his or her purpose and the condition of the physical world around them.

Keys can be used or made to unlock countless experiences when we do what it takes to become aware of what immediate situations require of us. The universe is constantly providing us with lessons and opportunities for advancement disguised as trials and tests.

Love is the most powerful force in our universe and can be seen and felt in the form of light.

Levels reveal themselves to us when we do the necessary work to qualify for them. The highest of these exist at our center and the lowest at our parameters or when we give power over to things and people outside of ourselves. There is no end to how far they can reach in either direction.

Magnetism is the byproduct of the pressure mediation that preceded it. It is essential to all forms of manifestation and

Measurement is necessary when it comes to making things right and exact. A specific amount of substances must be put into formulas to make them work the way they are meant to and if too much or too little is used then the outcome will be other than what was anticipated. The human body is highly intelligent and innately knows the proper amounts of nutrients to send to a cell or how much pain to produce when it needs us to tend to an issue.

Mitochondria are generally described as the powerhouses of the cells. Their origin is cosmic and we have a sort of symbiotic relationship with them. Science is constantly unraveling how significant they are in our everyday life but especially when it comes to improving our states of health. We will cover more on Mitochondria in *"Make The Hood Health Again Vol. 2"* and in our *Solar Powered Sunday* presentations.

New manifestations are always being created in the eternal present moment. The power of now unavoidably makes new things possible. What we call new has its origin in what our ancestors referred to as the waters of nu. Familiarize yourself with the ancient teachings found in Kemet/Egypt in order to get a better grasp of modern day terms.

Nutrients come in all types of forms and supply the body with what it needs in order for us to function correctly. Many of them can be produced naturally when we have adequate levels of sunlight and others must be consumed from various sources in nature.

Optimization is neglected by most as we tend to become satisfied with just feeling good or just normal after relieving pain or suffering from disease phenomena. Human body optimization is attainable if we make it point to change things at the causal level and push ourselves to the limit with the same level of intensity that we once perpetuated our bad habits.

Pressure is the language of Mother Nature. She doesn't care about how bad we desire to be healthy or how many times we think about doing better. She responds to pressure only whether it be physically or spiritually.

Rotation is what allows for us to experience the totality of a thing. In this text we witness it as the earth turns on its axis and as the Sun moves around larger stellar forces. It is significant because reaching true states of health requires for us to deal with our selves as a complete being and not exclusively in compartments unless they are all address and work together as a united force.

Spirituality put plain and simple is your relationship with the universe in and around you. Keeping in mind that everything is essentially made up of spirit we find it important to be mindful in how we deal with all things that we come into contact with and all things that our personal choices may end up having an effect on. The world inside of us is no less important than that which we se when opening our eyes each day. Even though all things are relevant to a degree, the world inside of us should be made a priority as it is home to all of the causes that we create. Spirituality has to less to do with wearing dashikis or crystals and more to do with being wise about how we manage the energy in and around us. Remember that where attention is energy is also present and that energy obeys and adjusts itself according to what we choose to concentrate on. We can shift our circumstances and how situations impact us simply by modifying our awareness and perception of the said event or situation at hand.

Time is the movement of magnetic fields. It is common now to hear that time is an illusion or a man made concept. Time can also be understood as the movement of the celestial spheres and can be used as a tool to help us measure how we distribute our energy throughout a lifetime.

Universe is derived from "uni" meaning one and verse meaning communication. There is only one cosmic conversation occurring. This conversation however involves all of the voices of the beings that exist as well as echoes from those who have already existed and inklings from those who have yet to be born.

Vibration is responsible for everything in the universe. Everything in existence has its own rate of vibration. We heal by restoring things back to their original rate and state of vibration.

Weather is determined by the collective consciousness and emotions of a group of people. While it is typically thought to change according to atmospheric conditions, we must keep in mind that all denser forms of matter including water and air are subject to our mental activities.

You are the concretization of the creator of the universe.

Zodiac is newer term referring to the circle of constellations that the Sun appears to travel thru as we circumambulate around it during the course of a year.

Thank you for allowing us to be a part of your journey back to wholeness! Remember you are your own project at the end of the day. Listen to others and study ardently but never stop listening to that inner voice of discernment to see what resonates with you.

Follow Asa Locket: www.asameansdoctor.com

@asameansdoctor - Instagram

@asalockett5 - Twitter

Follow Rafa Wright: www.neighborhood-grocery.com

@fairo_rafa – Instagram, Twitter, Fanbase, Tik Tok